T0259355

Pediatric Foot Deformities

Editor

PATRICK A. DEHEER

CLINICS IN PODIATRIC MEDICINE AND SURGERY

www.podiatric.theclinics.com

Consulting Editor
THOMAS ZGONIS

October 2013 • Volume 30 • Number 4

ELSEVIER

1600 John F. Kennedy Boulevard • Suite 1800 • Philadelphia, Pennsylvania, 19103-2899

http://www.theclinics.com

CLINICS IN PODIATRIC MEDICINE AND SURGERY Volume 30, Number 4
October 2013 ISSN 0891-8422, ISBN-13: 978-0-323-22716-2

Editor: Patrick Manley

Clinics in Podiatric Medicine and Surgery (ISSN 0891-8422) is published quarterly by Elsevier Inc., 360 Park Avenue South, New York, NY 10010-1710. Months of issue are January, April, July, and October. Business and Editorial Offices: 1600 John F. Kennedy Blvd., Ste. 1800, Philadelphia, PA 19103-2899. Customer Service Office: 3251 Riverport Lane, Maryland Heights, MO 63043. Periodicals postage paid at New York, NY and additional mailing offices. Subscription prices are $292.00 per year for US individuals, $410.00 per year for US institutions, $148.00 per year for US students and residents, $350.00 per year for Canadian individuals, $508.00 for Canadian institutions, $415.00 for international individuals, $508.00 per year for international institutions and $208.00 per year for Canadian and foreign students/residents. To receive student/resident rate, orders must be accompanied by name of affiliated institution, date of term, and the signature of program/residency coordinator on institution letterhead. Orders will be billed at individual rate until proof of status is received. Foreign air speed delivery is included in all Clinics subscription prices. All prices are subject to change without notice. POSTMASTER: Send address changes to Clinics in Podiatric Medicine and Surgery, Elsevier Health Sciences Division, Subscription Customer Service, 3251 Riverport Lane, Maryland Heights, MO 63043. **Customer Service: 1-800-654-2452 (US). From outside of the US, call 314-447-8871. Fax: 314-447-8029. E-mail: JournalsCustomerService-usa@elsevier.com (for print support); JournalsOnlineSupport-usa@elsevier.com (for online support).**

Reprints. For copies of 100 or more of articles in this publication, please contact the Commercial Reprints Department, Elsevier Inc., 360 Park Avenue South, New York, NY 10010-1710. Tel.: 212-633-3874; Fax: 212-633-3820; E-mail: reprints@elsevier.com.

Clinics in Podiatric Medicine and Surgery is covered in MEDLINE/PubMed (Index Medicus) and EMBASE/Excerpta Medica.

Printed and bound by CPI Group (UK) Ltd, Croydon, CR0 4YY

Transferred to digital print 2012

CLINICS IN PODIATRIC MEDICINE AND SURGERY

CONSULTING EDITOR
THOMAS ZGONIS, DPM, FACFAS

Contributors

CONSULTING EDITOR

THOMAS ZGONIS, DPM, FACFAS
Associate Professor, Externship and Fellowship Director in Reconstructive Foot and Ankle Surgery, Division of Podiatric Medicine and Surgery, Department of Orthopaedic Surgery, University of Texas Health Science Center at San Antonio, San Antonio, Texas

EDITOR

PATRICK A. DEHEER, DPM, FACFAS, FASPS
President, Wound Care Haiti; Podiatrist, Hoosier Foot and Ankle, LLC, Franklin, Indiana

AUTHORS

PATRICK AGNEW, DPM, FACFAS, FACFAP
Director of Podiatry Education, Eastern Virginia Medical School, Norfolk, Virginia

NATHAN COLEMAN, DPM
Resident, Podiatric Medicine and Surgery Residency, Trinity Regional Medical Center, UnityPoint Foot and Ankle, Fort Dodge, Iowa

PAUL DAYTON, DPM, MS, FACFAS
Director, Podiatric Medicine and Surgery Residency, Trinity Regional Medical Center, UnityPoint Foot and Ankle, Fort Dodge, Iowa

PATRICK A. DEHEER, DPM, FACFAS, FASPS
President, Wound Care Haiti; Podiatrist, Hoosier Foot and Ankle, LLC, Franklin, Indiana

LAWRENCE A. DIDOMENICO, DPM, FACFAS
Director of Fellowship Training; Adjunct Professor, Kent State College of Podiatric Medicine,Ohio; Chief Section Director, St. Elizabeth Hospital, Youngstown, Ohio

RAMY FAHIM, DPM
Fellow, Ankle and Foot Care Centers/ Kent State University College of Podiatric Medicine, Ohio; St. Elizabeth Hospital, Youngstown, Ohio

MINDI FEILMEIER, DPM, FACFAS
Assistant Professor, College of Podiatric Medicine and Surgery, Des Moines University, Des Moines, Iowa

MICHAEL E. GRAHAM, DPM, FACFAS, FAENS
Founder and Director, Graham International Implant Institute, Macomb, Michigan

EDWIN HARRIS, DPM, FACFAS
Clinical Associate Professor, Department of Orthopaedics and Rehabilitation, Stritch School of Medicine, Loyola University Chicago, Maywood; Private Practice, Westchester, Illinois

ALISON M. JOSEPH, DPM
Podiatry Attending, Department of Podiatry, University Hospital, Newark, New Jersey

IRENE K. LABIB, DPM
Podiatry Chief Resident, Department of Podiatry, University Hospital, Newark, New Jersey

RON RADUCANU, DPM
Private Practice, Philadelphia, Pennsylvania

JOHN J. STAPLETON, DPM, FACFAS
Associate, Foot and Ankle Surgery, VSAS Orthopaedics and Chief of Podiatric Surgery, Lehigh Valley Hospital, Allentown; Clinical Assistant Professor of Surgery, Penn State College of Medicine, Hershey, Pennsylvania

ZACHARY THOMAS, DPM
Resident, Heritage Medical Center, Beaver, Pennsylvania

HAROLD JACOB PIETER VAN BOSSE, MD
Department of Orthopaedic Surgery, Shriners Hospital for Children; Associate Professor of Orthopaedic Surgery, Department of Orthopaedic Surgery, Temple University, Philadelphia, Pennsylvania

AARON M. WARNOCK, DPM
Podiatrist, Hoosier Foot and Ankle, LLC, Franklin, Indiana

Contents

Foreword: Pediatric Foot Deformities   xi

Thomas Zgonis

Preface: Pediatric Foot Deformities   xiii

Patrick A. DeHeer

Lower Extremity Pediatric History and Physical Examination   461

Aaron M. Warnock, Ron Raducanu, and Patrick A. DeHeer

Although the pediatric foot and ankle examination is essentially similar to that of the adult patient, there are subtle differences unique to a child's examination. The unique findings are discussed in this article based on the following: weight-bearing examination, gait evaluation, non–weight-bearing examination, vascular examination, neurologic examination, and dermatologic examination for pediatric patients. A comprehensive overview is provided; however, other challenges presented in evaluating children include management of a child's parents and a child's temperament. The setting for an examination and a child's mood must be taken into consideration to ensure a successful outcome.

Pediatric Forefoot Pathology   479

Ramy Fahim, Zachary Thomas, and Lawrence A. DiDomenico

Surgical management of the pediatric forefoot often brings challenges to the foot and ankle surgeon. It requires a thorough understanding of the pathologic abnormality and underlying causes involved, which include the contributing genetic conditions. Albeit most of the deformities carry a rare level of incidence, they do however have a significant level of psychological component and stress on the pediatric patient. The goals of managing those pathologic abnormalities are ultimately to improve function while achieving a cosmetically acceptable outcome. The common forefoot pathologic abnormalities in the pediatric population are reviewed with an added focus toward management of forefoot trauma.

Pediatric First Ray Deformities   491

Patrick Agnew

Pediatric first ray deformities may present in many ways similar to those effecting adults. However, these patients are not adults. Management of the patient and the deformity necessitates special consideration of timing, the patient's general health, techniques, and perhaps goals. Any simple broad brush approach to the care of these patients will certainly result in both undertreatment and overtreatment. The proper care of these patients is an ongoing process of appropriate management tailored to the patient's needs, deformities, and developmental age. Proper adherence to these recommendations can improve the patient's quality of life.

Pediatric Heel Pain   503

Alison M. Joseph and Irene K. Labib

Heel pain is a common complaint among young children and adolescents. It has many causes, including trauma, overuse injuries, and tumors, and therefore a thorough clinical examination is warranted. This article outlines some common causes of pediatric heel pain.

Treatment of the Neglected and Relapsed Clubfoot   513

Harold Jacob Pieter van Bosse

Treatment of the neglected and the relapsed clubfoot is one of the most controversial topics in pediatric foot care. This article reviews the breadth of treatment options for practicing podiatrists or orthopedists with a specialty in complex clubfoot treatment. Discussion includes the appropriate circumstances for the use of the different procedures presented and the author's preferred treatment algorithm, based on 15 years of treating neglected, relapsed, and nonidiopathic clubfeet.

The Intoeing Child: Etiology, Prognosis, and Current Treatment Options   531

Edwin Harris

Intoeing, a common entrance complaint in infants, toddlers, and young children, is best defined as internal rotation of the long axis of the foot to the line of progression. Intoeing may be caused by primary deformities within the foot, issues with tibial torsion, and femoral antetorsion (anteversion). Problems within the foot include hallux varus, metatarsus adductus, talipes equinovarus, and pes cavus, each of which has specific treatments available. Treatment must be individualized, and the risks and complications weighed against the predictable morbidity of intoeing.

Congenital Talotarsal Joint Displacement and Pes Planovalgus: Evaluation, Conservative Management, and Surgical Management   567

Michael E. Graham

The diagnosis of and preferred treatment regimens for pediatric flatfoot, a complex and ambiguous deformity, continues to be debated. Incongruence of the talotarsal joint, whether flexible or rigid, is always present in pes planovalgus. However, it is important to note that talotarsal dislocation can occur without a flatfoot. The displacement of the talus on the hindfoot bones serves as the apex of the deformity. External measures, such as conservative care, are limited in providing correction to this internal deformity. Extraosseous talotarsal stabilization provides a minimally invasive internal option that should be considered before more radical surgical intervention is decided upon.

Principles of Management of Growth Plate Fractures in the Foot and Ankle   583

Paul Dayton, Mindi Feilmeier, and Nathan Coleman

Providers treating pediatric injuries must understand the properties of the pediatric skeleton and be sensitive to the psychological and social expectations of patients and their families. Immediate needs must be addressed, and the long-term prognosis must be explained. Detailed understanding of fracture mechanism and fracture patterns is essential for diagnosis and treatment. The provider must remain vigilant for changes in the osseous and soft tissue structures during treatment. Failure to recognize signs of growth interruption and changes in position may lead to functional abnormalities. This article presents an overview of pediatric growth plate injury management.

Current Concepts and Techniques in Foot and Ankle Surgery

Simultaneous Surgical Repair of a Tibialis Anterior Tendon Rupture and Diabetic Charcot Neuroarthropathy of the Midfoot: A Case Report   **599**

John J. Stapleton

The combination of simultaneous rupture of a tibialis anterior tendon and Charcot neuroarthropathy of the midfoot in a diabetic patient is a rare and challenging condition that can lead to major complications if not addressed appropriately. This article discusses a tibialis anterior tendon rupture that may have developed before or after the incidence of the diabetic Charcot neuroarthropathy midfoot deformity and raises awareness to potential spontaneous tendon ruptures that may be associated with the diabetic Charcot foot.

Erratum   **605**

Erratum   **607**

Index   **609**

CLINICS IN PODIATRIC MEDICINE AND SURGERY

FORTHCOMING ISSUES

January 2014
Medical and Surgical Management of the Diabetic Foot and Ankle
Peter A. Blume, DPM, *Editor*

April 2014
Hallux Abducto Valgus Surgery
Babek Baravarian, DPM, *Editor*

July 2014
Adult Acquired Flatfoot Deformity
Alan R. Catanzariti, DPM and
Robert W. Mendicino, DPM, *Editors*

RECENT ISSUES

July 2013
Advances in Forefoot Surgery
Charles M. Zelen, DPM, *Editor*

April 2013
Revision Total Ankle Replacement
Thomas S. Roukis, DPM, *Editor*

January 2013
Primary Total Ankle Replacement
Thomas S. Roukis, DPM, *Editor*

Foreword

Pediatric Foot Deformities

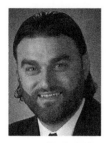

Thomas Zgonis, DPM, FACFAS
Consulting Editor

This edition of *Clinics in Podiatric Medicine and Surgery* is focused entirely on the conservative and surgical management of pediatric foot deformities. A great variety of pathology including congenital and acquired conditions are well covered by the experienced invited authors and guest editor, Dr DeHeer. Topics such as congenital pes planovalgus deformity, hallux varus, and metatarsus adductus are described in detail along with a complete and thorough evaluation of the lower extremity. Pediatric heel pain, treatment of the neglected clubfoot, as well as pediatric traumatic injuries are also emphasized and reviewed in detail.

In addition, I would like to thank again all of the invited authors, guest editors, editorial board members, and *Clinics in Podiatric Medicine and Surgery* managerial leadership for their ongoing efforts in providing guidance and excellence in the entire publication process. Last, I would also like to emphasize the "Current Concepts and Techniques in Foot and Ankle Surgery" section at the end of each *Clinics in Podiatric Medicine and Surgery* issue, which encourages submissions from a variety of research articles, case reports, or surgical techniques.

Thomas Zgonis, DPM, FACFAS
Associate Professor
Externship and Fellowship Director in Reconstructive Foot and Ankle Surgery
Division of Podiatric Medicine and Surgery
Department of Orthopaedic Surgery
University of Texas Health Science Center at San Antonio
7703 Floyd Curl Drive MSC 7776
San Antonio, Texas 78229, USA

E-mail address:
zgonis@uthscsa.edu

Clin Podiatr Med Surg 30 (2013) xi
http://dx.doi.org/10.1016/j.cpm.2013.08.002
0891-8422/13/$ – see front matter © 2013 Elsevier Inc. All rights reserved.
podiatric.theclinics.com

Preface

Pediatric Foot Deformities

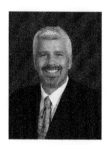

Patrick A. DeHeer, DPM, FACFAS, FASPS
Editor

The evaluation and management of pediatric foot and ankle deformities are of vital importance regardless of the foot and ankle expert's practice makeup. The clear pathway of deformity seen in the child leads to pathology into adulthood, so if your practice is primarily adult based or if a large percentage is pediatric, it is imperative to have an understanding of pediatric deformities and pathologies. If an asymptomatic pediatric deformity is treated appropriately, typical associated adult pathology may be prevented. This role of adult preventative care when a deformity is present in childhood is an often ignored component of care.

With this *Clinics in Podiatric Medicine and Surgery*, I have attempted to cover some of the more common pediatric pathologies. The list of topics is wide-ranging and the authors are respected experts and well-published. One of my goals was to bring together the pediatric orthopedics and pediatric podiatric medicine. I was able to accomplish this goal somewhat, but not to the extent I had hoped. A joining of the minds from both groups can only benefit the pediatric patients entrusted to our care and I hope to see more collaboration in the future.

I would like to personally thank those that contributed to this volume as well as my wife, Erika Jagger DeHeer, for her support during the editing of this edition.

Patrick A. DeHeer, DPM, FACFAS, FASPS
Hoosier Foot & Ankle, LLC
Wound Care Haiti
1159 West Jefferson Street
Suite 204
Franklin, IN 46131, USA

E-mail address:
padeheer@sbcglobal.net

Clin Podiatr Med Surg 30 (2013) xiii
http://dx.doi.org/10.1016/j.cpm.2013.08.001
0891-8422/13/$ – see front matter © 2013 Elsevier Inc. All rights reserved.

Lower Extremity Pediatric History and Physical Examination

Aaron M. Warnock, DPM[a], Ron Raducanu, DPM[b],
Patrick A. DeHeer, DPM[a],*

KEYWORDS

- Foot and ankle examination • Pediatric examination • Weight-bearing examination
- Non–weight-bearing examination

KEY POINTS

- Although the pediatric foot and ankle examination is essentially similar to that of the adult patient, there are subtle differences that are unique to a child's examination and it is of utmost importance that the provider is able to recognize these differences.
- The physical examination should be organized by topographic considerations; head, shoulders, upper extremities, hips, knees, and then feet.
- Once the provider has recognized any pathology in the pediatric patient the provider must outline a detailed and concise treatment plan to ensure compliance by the patient and his or her family.
- Failure to recognize subtle pathological changes during the pediatric evaluation may lead to devastating, long-term abnormalities.

Although the pediatric foot and ankle examination is essentially similar to that of the adult patient, there are subtle differences that are unique to a child's examination. The unique findings are discussed in this article based on the following: weight-bearing examination, gait evaluation, non–weight-bearing examination, vascular examination, neurologic examination, and dermatologic examination for pediatric patients. A comprehensive overview is provided of this examination; however, there are other challenges presented in evaluating children, including management of a child's parents and a child's temperament. The setting for an examination and a child's mood must be taken into consideration prior to undertaking an examination to ensure a successful outcome.

WEIGHT-BEARING GAIT EVALUATION AND NORMAL DEVELOPMENT

The gait assessment begins with a patient walking with and without shoes; visual observation of whether the gait pattern is normal, antalgic, or indicative of neuromuscular disease should be noted. The examination should be organized by topographic

[a] Hoosier Foot & Ankle, LLC, 1159 West Jefferson Street, Suite 204, Franklin, IN 46131, USA;
[b] Private Practice, 123 Chestnut Street, Suite 201 Philadelphia, PA 19106, USA
* Corresponding author.
E-mail address: padeheer@sbcglobal.net

Clin Podiatr Med Surg 30 (2013) 461–478
http://dx.doi.org/10.1016/j.cpm.2013.07.008   **podiatric.theclinics.com**
0891-8422/13/$ – see front matter © 2013 Elsevier Inc. All rights reserved.

considerations; head, shoulders, upper extremities, hips, knees, and then feet. The head should be rectus in the frontal and sagittal planes without any left, right, anterior, or posterior deviation. Frontal plane deviation can indicate a neurologic defect or any neuromuscular disease that affects the extraocular muscles. A positive head tilt can also be contributed to a limb length discrepancy; this can be measured by placing a tape measure at the anterior superior iliac spine and measuring to the floor. The head tilts toward the short side when compensated and toward the long side when un-compensated. If there is deviation in the sagittal plane, the authors most commonly see kyphosis and neurologic problems as the underlying cause (Spencer S. DPM, un-published data, 2011).[1]

The shoulders are then evaluated and should show no deviation in the frontal, sagittal, and transverse planes. Shoulder deviation in the frontal plane can indicate scoliosis or a limb length discrepancy. Poor posture and kyphosis are attributed to any sagittal plane deviation (Spencer S. DPM, unpublished data, 2011).[1]

The upper extremity arm swing should be symmetric when observed in the frontal plane. Circumduction of the arm and wide swinging of the extremity may indicate possible neurologic problems. Valmassy[1] states classically that if there is a limb length discrepancy, the long leg circumducts to prevent the toes from dragging, resulting in a greater arm swing on the short leg side. Arm swing in the sagittal plane should encompass a two-thirds anterior swing to the body's midline and a one-third posterior arm swing to the body's midline. If abduction of the arm is present, this suggests an uncompensated or partially compensated limb length discrepancy (Spencer S. DPM, unpublished data, 2011).[1]

The trunk and pelvis should exhibit symmetric rotation during the gait cycle in all planes. The iliac crests should be equal and level with one another on the frontal plane. Any difference is likely due to a limb length discrepancy. A common disorder of the hips and pelvis is Trendelenburg gait. Valmassy states that when standing on one leg, the center of gravity is brought over the weight-bearing foot by the gluteal muscles on that side, tilting the pelvis. The pelvic tilt results in elevation of the buttocks on the other side. The bending of the trunk toward the side of the supporting limb during stance phase is known as lateral trunk bending of Trendelenburg gait. The purpose of this movement is to reduce the forces in the abductor muscles and the hip joint during single support stance. A positive Trendelenburg sign appears when the buttock on the non–weight-bearing side fails to rise due to weakness of the gluteus medius muscle (Spencer S. DPM, unpublished data, 2011)[1] (seen in **Fig. 1**).

Concerning the knee, the patella should be internally rotated and then externally rotated until it is straight during midstance. If the authors see an internally rotated knee, this may indicate an in-toe type of gait. An in-toe type of gait shows a negative angle of gait or adduction of the foot in the transverse plane relative to the line of progression. The apex of the deformity can be at any level of the lower extremity. Acetabular anteversion of the pelvis, femoral anteversion of the hip, genu varum, tibial torsion of the leg, metatarsus adductus, and clubfoot are examples of different apexes of deformity.[2–4] During the gait cycle, evaluate if the knees are on the frontal plane. If in-toeing is evident and the knees are in the frontal plane, then the deformity exists in the foot. If the knees are not on the in the frontal plane, then the deformity exists in the hip. CT scans and computer-aided models provide the most accurate measurements of acetabular and femoral anteversion if coxa vara is suspected.

The gait pattern for early walkers is much different than that of adults because they are continuing to mature and have a different location of their center of gravity. Adults tend to have a center of gravity located anterior to the second sacral vertebrae. Beginning walkers' center of gravity is located above the umbilicus to the pubic symphysis.

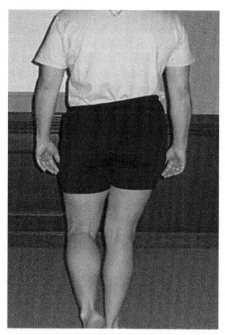

Fig. 1. Trendelenburg gait. Note the hip drop on the non–weight-bearing side.

Beginning walkers' step cadence is high because they have reduced stride length with a wide base of gait due to an externally rotated hip. The calcaneus is constantly everted for added stability. Clinicians should also note a flatfoot strike with elbows fixed in flexion, and arms abducted.

During ambulation, note if toe walking is present (seen in **Fig. 2**). Toe walking is commonly seen in early walkers due to the ankle allowing 20° to 30° of dorsiflexion. This dorsiflexion decreases to approximately 10° in adults. Abnormalities in this progression are most commonly seen as gastrocnemius, soleus, or gastrosoleal equinus; bony/cartilaginous ankle block; pseudoequinus; or cavus foot. Ankle equinus is a routine encounter for podiatrists and is prevalent in the general population. Cass

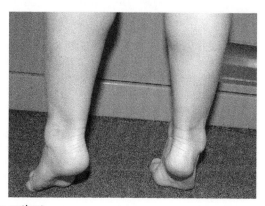

Fig. 2. Toe walking patient.

and Canasta[5] state, however, that lack of dorsiflexion may be found begining prox-imally with tight hip flexor muscles and can be identified with a Thomas test. In a su-pine examination, flexion of one hip to the torso should allow the contralateral hip to remain in a fully extended position. Rising of the contralateral leg after this flexion ma-neuver on the opposite limb is a clinical sign of hip flexor tightness. Next, children should be checked for tightness of the hamstring muscles on straight-leg raise, popli-teal angle, or toe-touching examination. Distally, the appropriate clinical examination is the Silfverskiöld test. In 1924, Silfverskiöld divided spastic equinus contracture into 2 groups, 1 of which is passively correctable by flexion of the knee to a right angle. Silfverskiöld performed his test to assess dorsiflexion of a neutral foot on the lower leg with the knee extended (testing gastrocnemius) and knee flexed (testing soleus or bony block)[6] (demonstrated in **Figs. 3** and **4**).

While stationary, evaluate the lower leg for genu varum and genu valgum. Genu varum is measured by the long axis of the distal one-third of the leg with a line perpen-dicular to the ground. Genu varum is widely recognized up to 2 years of age and typi-cally resolves without treatment. If it does not resolve at an early age, it is not benign. During the adult years, premature and eccentric stress on the knee may result in medial meniscal tears, tibiofemoral subluxation, articular cartilage attrition, and arthrosis of the medial compartment of the knee.[2–4] At times, genu recurvatum may be observed with genu varum; 5° to 10° is considered normal. Patients should have no recurvatum at age 6 years.[2–4]

Genu valgum (demonstrated in **Fig. 3**) is observed in association with an outward torsion of the femur, tibia, or both. A normal variant of the disorder in toddlers typically is symmetric and pain-free, but it should resolve spontaneously by the time the child is aged 6 years.[2–4] If the valgus is unilateral or symptomatic, referral to an orthopedist and radiographic evaluation are warranted.

Tibial torsion is the lateral twist of the long axis of the tibia. When stationary, this angle is typically measured by the malleolar position by the use of goniometers, tracto-graphs, or other angle-measuring devices. Malleolar position is typically 5° less than actual tibial torsion. At birth, the malleolar position should be 0 and increase 2° to 3° every year, averaging 20° in adults.[2–4]

While still stationary, the resting calcaneal stance position is evaluated with patients standing in a normal base of gait on a hard level surface. Clinicians measure the angle of the bisection of the calcaneus and the supporting surface. Sobel and colleagues[7]

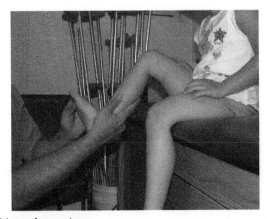

Fig. 3. Silfverskiöld test for equinus.

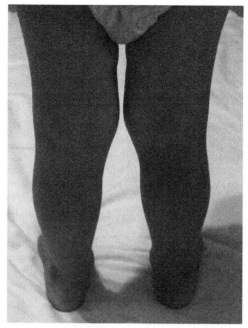

Fig. 4. Genu valgum of a 2-year-old patient.

measured 88 adults and 124 children, ranging in age from 5 to 36 years. The mean relaxed calcaneal stance position for adults was 6.07° valgus. The mean relaxed calcaneal stance position for children was 5.6° valgus. They stated that was no significant difference between the relaxed calcaneal stance positions of adults and children and that the children's relaxed calcaneal stance position did not correlate with age, height, or weight and did not decrease with age to the theoretic normal value of $0° \pm 2°$, as postulated by Root and colleagues. For the neutral calcaneal stance, position the subtalar joint (STJ) in neutral position. The angle is again measured. Neutral calcaneal stance position places the STJ in maximum congruency. This essentially gives the total rearfoot deformity that is present compared with the resting calcaneal stance position.

NON–WEIGHT-BEARING BIOMECHANICAL EXAMINATION

During the non–weight-bearing pediatric examination, it is important to evaluate patients' joint positions and range of motion. If restriction of joint motion is observed, it must be determined if it is due to spastic diseases, bony or cartilaginous blocks, congenital fusions, tarsal coalitions, muscle shortening, or contractures.

Orthopedic Examination of the Hip

The pediatric hip alignment must also be evaluated. A patient's angle of declination or antetorsion of the femur is the measured from the bisection of the long axis of the femoral neck and the condyles in the coronal plane. This is best evaluated clinically using the Ryder test, which places the greater trochanter of the femur parallel to the frontal plane of a child while lying supine. With the proximal segment maintained in this position parallel to the frontal plane, the transcondylar axis of the femur is evaluated at the level of the knee joint. At 1 year, the angle should be 39°; at 10 years, 24°; at age 21, 16°; and in adults, 6°.[4]

A frequent encounter in many podiatry clinics is congenital hip dislocation. Congenital hip dislocation is variable and depends on many factors. Approximately 1 in 1000 children is born with a dislocated hip, and 10 in 1000 may have hip subluxation. Factors contributing to congenital hip dislocation include breech presentation, female gender, positive family history, firstborn status, and oligohydramnios. Intrauterine position, gender, race, and positive family history are the most important risk factors. The hip may be evaluated by use of the anchor sign, Galeazzi sign, Ortolani sign, or Barlow sign.[8–10]

The anchor sign is asymmetry of the thigh folds, and the gluteal and popliteal creases are seen in approximately 50% of all newborns and young infants.

The test for Galeazzi sign is performed by placing a child supine with hips and knees flexed (seen in **Fig. 5**). The affected side is lower than the nonaffected side.[8–10]

The test for Ortolani sign is performed with a baby supine with legs and hips flexed to 90°. The hips are examined one at a time by grasping the baby's thigh with the middle finger over the greater trochanter and then lifting and abducting the thigh to be examined while stabilizing the opposite thigh and pelvis (seen in **Fig. 6**). If hip is dislocated, the femoral head moves from a posterior position to a more anterior and distal position inside the acetabulum. The head relocating can be felt and it is described as a palpable click.[8–10]

The test for Barlow sign is performed when the hips are flexed to a right angle and the knees are fully flexed. Physicians place a middle finger over the greater trochanter with the thumb applied over the inner thigh opposite the position of the lesser trochanter. The thighs are then carried through midabduction while applying pressure backwards and outwards with the thumb. If the femoral head slips out over the posterior lip of the acetabulum and back again immediately when the pressure is released, the hip is unstable or dislocatable.[8–10]

The Barlow test is demonstrated in **Figs. 7–9**.

Orthopedic Examination of the Knee

Examination of the knee should begin with the patella. Tracking is assessed by observing the patella for smooth motion while the patient contracts the quadriceps muscle. The presence of crepitus should be noted during palpation of the patella.[11]

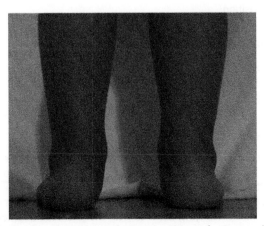

Fig. 5. Valgus attitude of resting calcaneal stance position of a 2-year-old patient.

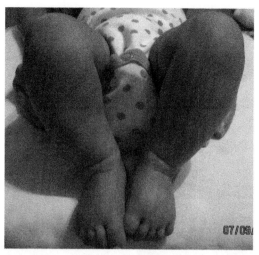

Fig. 6. Galeazzi test. Normal hip of 4-month-old patient. If the hip is dislocated, the affected side is lower.

A patellar apprehension test is then performed. With fingers placed at the medial aspect of the patella, the physician attempts to sublux the patella laterally. Both the superior and inferior patellar facets should be palpated, with the patella subluxed first medially and then laterally.[11] The vruciate ligaments of the knee should be evaluated. The anterior drawer tests the anterior cruciate ligament. The patient assumes a supine position with the knee flexed to 90°. The physician fixes the patient's foot in slight external rotation and then places the thumbs at the tibial tubercle with the fingers at the posterior calf. With the patient's hamstring muscles relaxed, the physician pulls anteriorly and assesses anterior displacement of the tibia (anterior drawer sign).[11] The Lachman test is another means of assessing the integrity of the anterior cruciate ligament. The test is performed with the patient in a supine position with the knee flexed to 30°. The physician stabilizes the distal femur with one hand, grasps the

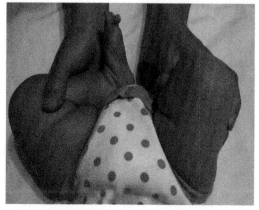

Fig. 7. Ortolani test. If the femoral head relocates with a palpable click, then the test is positive.

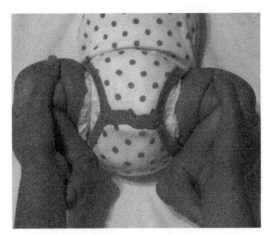

Fig. 8. Barlow test.

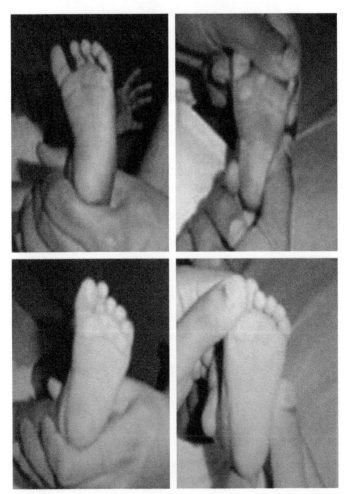

Fig. 9. Note the adducted foot. Technique for assessing flexibility of the deformity. Note the rearfoot is stabilized while the forefoot is abducted.

proximal tibia in the other hand, and then attempts to sublux the tibia anteriorly. Lack of a clear endpoint indicates a positive Lachman test.[11]

The posterior cruciate ligament is accessed with the posterior drawer test. The patient assumes a supine position with knees flexed to 90°. While standing at the side of the examination table, the physician looks for posterior displacement of the tibia. Next, the physician fixes the patient's foot in a neutral position rotation, positions thumbs at the tibial tubercle, and places fingers at the posterior calf. The physician then pushes posteriorly and assesses for posterior displacement of the tibia.[11]

The integrity of the collateral ligaments of the knee is assessed as well. The medial collateral ligament is accessed by placing one hand at the lateral aspect of the knee joint and the other hand at the medial aspect of the distal tibia; next, a valgus stress is applied to the knee with it fully extended and at 30° of flexion. The knee should be stable without any laxity at both positions. The lateral collateral ligament is tested with one hand at the medial aspect of the patient's knee and the other hand at the lateral aspect of the distal fibula with a varus stress at full extension and at 30° flexion.[11]

The ankle ligaments are tested with the anterior drawer test and the inversion stress test. The test is performed with the patient supine or sitting up with the knees flexed over the table's edge. One hand is held against the anterior tibia and the other hand grasps the posterior aspect of the heel. The foot is internally rotated a slight degree to relax the deltoid ligament. The ankle is placed in a neutral position. The calcaneus is then pulled forward while the tibia is stabilized simultaneously. In the event that the anterior talofibular ligament is compromised, the talus displaces anteriorly from beneath the tibia, and a dell may be appreciated in the skin of the anterolateral aspect of the ankle joint. Normal values for anterior displacement may range from 2.5 mm to 3 mm, and, in general, anterior displacement of the talus greater than 4 mm is considered a positive result.

Performing the stress inversion test is valuable in assessing combined laxity of the anterior talofibular and the calcaneofibular ligaments. An isolated rupture of the anterior talofibular ligament may result in a small increase in talar tilt. The stress inversion test is performed with one hand grasping the heel while the opposite hand stabilizes the medial aspect of the leg just above the malleoli. The rearfoot and ankle are then forcefully inverted. The normal value for talar tilt is 5° or less in manually stressed ankles.[12]

EXAMINATION OF THE FOOT
Metatarsus Adductus

McGlamry states that metatarsus adductus is a structural deformity in which the metatarsals are excessively adducted in relation to the lesser tarsus at the tarsometatarsal joints in the transverse plane. Metatarsus adductus leads to a gait that appears more adducted and causes increased lateral pressure on the metatarsal heads at propulsion. Patients with rigid types of this disorder may be unstable in the stance phase of gait. In more flexible foot types, compensation is often by STJ pronation, which occurs as the adducted foot is forced into a normal-last shoe. McGlamry states that the ARM (components of the pediatric evaluation: attitude, relationship, and movement) method of physical examination described by Ganley facilitates immediate appreciation of the metarsus adductus deformity. Metatarsus adductus essentially points the resting attitude of the foot medially, unless more a proximal deformity negates this appearance. Therefore, appreciation of the relationship of the forefoot to the rearfoot in all 3 cardinal planes is necessary.[13,14] A technique for assessing flexibility of metatarsus adductus is shown in **Fig. 10**. The rearfoot is stabilized by lateral pressure over the calcaneal cuboid joint and the forefoot is abducted.

Congenital Clubfoot

Clubfoot consists of 4 components: equinus, varus, adductus, and cavus deformity of the foot.[15,16] McGlamry states that Adams in 1866 was the first to postulate that the primary deforming force in clubfoot was an intrinsic talar deformity. These investigations stipulated that the intrinsic deformation of the talus lay within the malformed head and neck of the osseous precursor. Normally, the talar head and neck are adducted 15° to 20° in the transverse plane on the talar body. In the clubfoot, this angulation increases dramatically to 80° to 90°. In the sagittal plane, the talar head and neck are normally plantarflexed 25° to 30° in relation to the talar body. In clubfoot, this angulation is increased to 45° to 65°. Chief among the neuromuscular diseases and spinal abnormalities that may lead to a clubfoot are poliomyelitis, arthrogryphosis, meningitis, cerebral palsy, spina bifida, and myelomeningocele.[4] Previous trauma is also at the top of the list; such cases have been related to spinal trauma, neglected lower leg tendon rupture, and laceration, resulting in muscle imbalance. Volkmann contractures, burn contractures, and epiphyseal and malunited medial malleolar fractures are all too common causes of clubfoot. Clubfoot in developing countries is most often a result of direct sciatic trauma to an infant or child from a poorly placed gluteal injection.[17]

Staging

There is no agreed method of grading the severity of the clubfoot deformity or monitoring the natural history, but there is a reported need for such a classification, which should be reliable, reproducible, and feasible in a clinical setting and predict appropriate treatment. Dyer and Davis[18] devised a simple scoring system based on 6 clinical signs of contracture. Each is scored according to the following principle: 0, no abnormality; 0.5, moderate abnormality; and 1, severe abnormality.[15]

The 6 signs are separated into 3 related to the hindfoot (severity of the posterior crease, emptiness of the heel, and rigidity of the equinus) and 3 related to the midfoot (curvature of the lateral border of the foot, severity of the medial crease, and position of the lateral part of the head of the talus). Thus, each foot can receive a hindfoot score between 0 and 3, midfoot score between 0 and 3, and a total score between 0 and 6.[15,18]

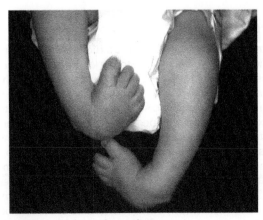

Fig. 10. Bilateral congenital clubfoot of an infant.

Dyer and Davis[18] reviewed Parani's method of scoring in 70 idiopathic clubfeet between February 2002 and May 2004. They found that there was a significant positive correlation between the initial Pirani score and number of casts required to correct the deformity. A foot scoring 4 or more is likely to require at least 4 casts, and a foot scoring less than 4 requires 3 or fewer. A foot with a hindfoot score of 2.5 or 3 has a 72% chance of requiring a tenotomy.[15] This scoring method is valuable not only to clinicians but also to parents. Parents whose children are starting Ponseti treatment are likely to enquire whether a tenotomy is required and how many casts their baby will require. The Pirani system answers this question. The Parani method is detailed in **Figs. 11–16**.

Rigid Flatfoot due to Coalition

A rigid flatfoot can have many causes; however, tarsal coalitions are by far the most frequently encountered cause. There are several proposed theories related to the cause of tarsal coalitions. Cass and colleagues[5] state that the most widely accepted is LeBouq's theory of failure of differentiation of embryonic mesenchymal tissue, believed to be a heritable autosomal dominant defect or an insult sustained in the first trimester of pregnancy. It is bilateral 50% to 80% of the time.[8] The investigators state that in their experience unilateral tarsal coalition is much more common than bilateral coalition. McGlamry states that there does not seem to be a gender predilection of tarsal coalitions, which is consistent with an autosomal dominant inheritance theory.[9] Cass states that calcaneonavicular and talocalcaneal coalitions make up 90% of coalitions. A talonavicular coalition is the third most common coalition, with fewer than 50 cases reported in the literature.[5] Limitation of STJ and midtarsal joint (MTJ) motion is common with tarsal coalition and is typically the most obvious clinical finding. Physicians can measure the number of degrees of STJ supination by fully inverting the calcaneus on the talus. A ratio of two-thirds supination to one-third pronation, with the total range of motion 30° (with 20° of inversion and 10° of eversion), should be seen.[19] If range of motion is lacking during the examination, clinicians must suspect a tarsal coalition.

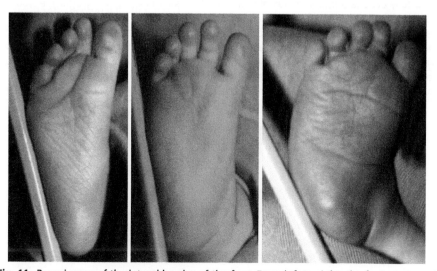

Fig. 11. Parani score of the lateral border of the foot. From left to right, the feet are scored 0, 0.5, and 1.0.

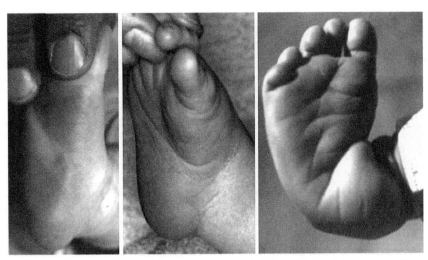

Fig. 12. Parani score of the medial heel crease. From left to right, the feet are scored 0, 0.5, and 1.0.

Flexible Flatfoot and Juvenile Hallux Abducto Valgus

A stepwise approach to evaluating pediatric flatfoot and juvenile hallux abducto valgus should be used by clinicians. The first ray must be evaluated for hypermobility. There should be equal excursion dorsally and plantarly to approximately (5 mm) of the first ray from a level equal with the second metatarsal when the STJ is in its neutral position and MTJ is maximally pronated. A hypermobile first ray may lead to juvenile hallux abducto valgus deformity or acquired pes planus. The first metatarsophalangeal joint should be evaluated for tracking and lateral deviation. Clinicians should note any prominent medial eminence to the first metatarsophalangeal joint and if painful on palpation. Radiographs can be taken to fully assess the severity of the deformity.

To fully assess a patient's flexible flatfoot, the patient is asked to perform a double heel rise test to evaluate the posterior tibial tendon function. Resting and neutral calcaneal stance positions are performed and each position is noted. In the mild flexible flatfoot, when the STJ is placed in a neutral position, the forefoot deformity should reduce with manipulation of the medial column (the toe test of Jack or the Hubscher maneuver). With the patient standing, external rotation of the leg and thigh with active or passive dorsiflexion of the great toe should result in restoration of the medial longitudinal

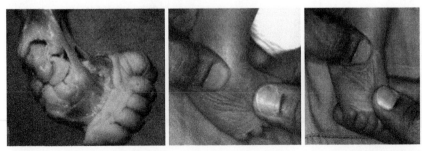

Fig. 13. Parani score of the talar head protrusion. From left to right, the feet are scored 0, 0.5, and 1.0.

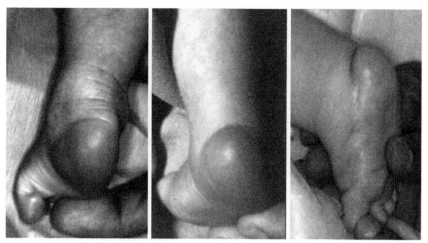

Fig. 14. Parani score of the posterior heel crease. From left to right, the feet are scored 0, 0.5, and 1.0.

arch and return of the heel to the vertical position.[20] The authors have observed that a pediatric flatfoot is normal until the age of 4.

Forefoot Varus and Forefoot Supinatus

Forefoot varus is a structural deformity showing inversion of the plantar plane of forefoot relative to rearfoot, when STJ is in neutral and MTJ is maximally pronated about both its axes. Forefoot varus is normal in early childhood and may exceed 10° but should not persist past 6 years of age. Forefoot supinatus is an acquired soft tissue deformity of longitudinal axis of MTJ, showing as inversion of forefoot relative to rearfoot when the STJ is in neutral position and MTJ is maximally pronated. As the hindfoot moves into a valgus alignment during gait, the forefoot inverts in reciprocal fashion to keep the metatarsals flat on the ground. Furthermore, as ligaments progressively rupture in the flatfoot, deformity occurs in the medial column, causing a dorsiflexion alignment. As the forefoot inverts on the rearfoot and as the medial column dorsiflexes, an acquired forefoot varus deformity occurs. To assess forefoot supinatus, evaluate the patient either supine or prone. In some cases, it may be more accurate to evaluate forefoot to rearfoot alignment with the patient in a prone position. The examination begins with the examiner holding the foot and grasping the heel and moving

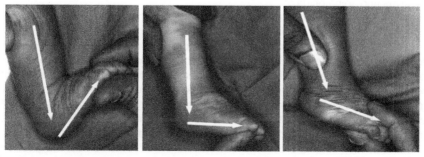

Fig. 15. Parani score of equinus. From left to right, the feet are scored 0, 0.5, and 1.0.

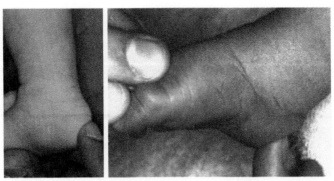

Fig. 16. Parani score of the empty heel. From left to right, the foot is scored 0 and 1.0.

the hindfoot to neutral or vertical. Then the frontal plane alignment of the forefoot to the rearfoot is evaluated, with the ankle dorsiflexed and then plantarflexed. As stated previously, up to 10° of forefoot varus is normal in patients up to 6 years of age. This component must be readily reducible on manual manipulation. When the STJ is placed in a neutral position, the forefoot deformity should reduce with manipulation of the medial column (the toe test of Jack or the Hubscher maneuver). With the patient standing, external rotation of the leg and thigh with active or passive dorsiflexion of the great toe should result in restoration of the medial longitudinal arch and return of the heel to the vertical position or the toe test of Jack may be used to assess the flexibility of the deformity. A fixed or rigid forefoot varus may be seen in pediatric patients and proper evaluation is needed to prevent long-term complications.[20]

Cavus Foot

McGlamry states that pes cavus is primarily a sagittal plane foot and ankle deformity in which the longitudinal arch is abnormally high. This may be considered either plantarflexion of the forefoot relative to the rearfoot or dorsiflexion of the rearfoot relative to the forefoot. The choice of reference is primarily a matter of perspective. The forefoot is primarily used, however, in defining pes cavus because deformity at this level tends to be the most dominant and more rigid component of the condition. Both rigid and flexible variants of pes cavus exist and can be classified as either congenital or acquired. Congenital conditions commonly associated with pes cavus include spina bifida and other myelodysplasias, familial degenerative nerve disease, hypertrophic interstitial neuropathy, cerebral palsy, muscular dystrophy, and congenital syphilis. A more significant correlation exists between pes cavus and scoliosis than between pes cavus and spina bifida.[21]

The initial premise is that pes cavus is primarily a sagittal plane deformity or a foot with an abnormally high longitudinal arch. Traditional terminology tends to describe the relationship of distal structures with more proximal structures. For this reason, pes cavus is defined as an excessive plantar declination of the forefoot, or part of the forefoot, on the rearfoot. This relationship from forefoot to rearfoot has traditionally been described as an anterior pes cavus. Pes cavus could also be described as an excessive dorsiflexion of the rearfoot on the forefoot. This has been termed, posterior pes cavus. This is actually a description of the same entity from 2 different perspectives. Theoretically and practically, anterior pes cavus and posterior pes cavus cannot exist without each other in order for the forefoot and rearfoot to contact the ground in gait.[21] Anterior equinus, also known as anterior cavus, is a deformity represented by a plantarflexed attitude of the forefoot or any of its component parts. This type of equinus may be subdivided into 4 types based on the apex of the deformity in the sagittal plane. These types include the aforementioned metatarsal equinus and forefoot equinus along with lesser tarsal equinus (an excessive plantarflexed deformity occurring in the lesser tarsal bones themselves) or a combination of these deformities. Although these types of anterior equinus occur in the foot and not in the ankle, an apparent or false ankle equinus mistakenly can be measured clinically. To explain, ankle equinus is a sagittal plane measurement of the bisection of the leg to the rearfoot. Inexperienced clinicians often falsely identify an ankle equinus in the anterior cavus foot if they measure the sagittal plane bisection of the leg to the forefoot. This allows any plantarflexion of the forefoot on the rearfoot to be included in the measurement. Identifying this problem and to avoid confusion, Whitney and Green[22] appropriately coined the term, pseudoequinus, to account for the false ankle equinus seen in an anterior cavus foot type (described previously). Thus, pseudoequinus is an angular relation of equinus of the forefoot to the leg in the sagittal plane without an equinus relation of the rearfoot to the leg in the sagittal plane Pseudoequinus is not a true ankle joint limitation but an excessive demand for ankle dorsiflexion created by forefoot equinus. This occurs because the entire foot must be dorsiflexed at the ankle to allow the heel of the foot with anterior equinus to reach the ground. Thus, ankle joint dorsiflexion is overtaxed to compensate for the anterior equinus deformity. If a clinician accepts that the deformity lies within the forefoot, then it is imperative to perform the Coleman block test. The Coleman block test indicates if there is enough range of motion of the STJ to invert to allow the heel to become perpendicular to the ground to accommodate for the forefoot valgus.[21]

To perform the Coleman block test, patients stand with their heel and the lateral side of their forefoot on a 1-inch block, so that the medial side of the forefoot (ie the first metatarsal head) is on the floor next to the block. If their heel has now corrected to a neutral position, this means they have a mobile hindfoot and the hindfoot is being forced into inversion (varus) by the platerflexed first metatarsal. If their hindfoot does not correct to a neutral alignment, the inversion is not just due to the plantarflexed first metatarsal. Clinicians should then look for other causes, such as fixed hindfoot inversion or tibialis posterior spasticity.

Neurologic Examination

A thorough neurologic examination should be performed on every pediatric patient. Patients should be evaluated for any signs of an upper motor neuron lesion or lower motor neuron lesion. Clinicians must be able to differentiate between the 2. Typically, upper motor neuron lesions manifest themselves as exaggerated tendon reflexes, hyperreflexia, and increase in muscle tone due to clonus, and the entire limb typically is affected. Lower motor neuron lesions typically present as a loss of tendon reflexes, muscle wasting, lack of tone, or flaccidity and usually only certain muscle groups are affected due to the antagonistic muscle group dominating. Conditions that are seen with upper motor neuron lesions are cerebral palsy due to anoxia a birth, cerebral vascular accident, Friedreich ataxia, spinal injury, amyotrophic lateral sclerosis, vitamin B_{12} deficiency, multiple sclerosis, and late stages of syringomyelia. Conditions seen that are seen with lower motor lesions are poliomyelitis, spina bifida, Charcot-Marie-tooth disease, injury to the lower motor neuron from trauma, and Brown-Séquard syndrome. The lower extremity neurologic examination should begin by trying to elicit a deep tendon reflex. The deep tendon reflexes are graded on a 4-point scale: 0 = absent despite reinforcement, 1 = present only with reinforcement, 2 = normal, 3 = increased but normal, and 4 = markedly hyperactive, with clonus. The patellar reflex (L2–L4) is performed by slightly lifting up of the leg under the knee and tapping the patellar tendon with a reflex hammer; there should be a reflex contraction of the quadriceps muscle. The ankle reflex (S1) is performed by slightly externally rotating the hip and gently dorsiflexing the foot and tapping the Achilles tendon; there should be a reflex contraction of the gastrocnemius.[23] When the reflexes are absent, eliciting it after reinforcement using the Jendrassik maneuver should be tried. The Jendrassik maneuver is wherein a patient flexes both sets of fingers into a hook-like form and interlocks those sets of fingers together, and a clinician then tries to elicit the patellar reflex again. The maneuver may prevent patients from consciously inhibiting or influencing their response to the hammer.[24–26] Clinicians must also realize that infantile reflexes show some variability compared with those of older children. Kumar and colleagues[27] studied 1281 children from age 1 to 12 months and found that the extensor plantar response was found in 79.4% of the patients up to age 6 months and 32% percent of the patients continued to have an extensor response (positive Babinski sign) to age 12 months. Clinicians must also evaluate the posterior column, lateral spinothalamic, and anterior spinothalamic tract, which is routinely accomplished with a tuning fork, sharp and dull instrument, and a Semmes-Weinstein 5.07 monofilament, respectively.

Vascular Examination

The dorsalis pedis pulse is typically located between the extensor hallucis longus and extensor digitorum longus tendons, just proximal and lateral to the dorsal prominence of the first metatarsal base and medial cuneiform. The posterior tibial pulse is palpable behind the medial malleolus, approximately one-third of the distance to the medial border of the Achilles tendon. If pulses are weak or absent, a more comprehensive vascular evaluation is warranted, especially if surgery is considered or if a patient has an open wound. Palpation should be done using the fingertips and intensity of the pulse graded on a scale of 0 to 4: 0 indicates no palpable pulse, 2 normal pulse, and 4 a bounding pulse. This evaluation may include pulse volume recordings with toe pressures or transcutaneous oxygen levels.[28]

Dermatologic Examination

Assess patients for ingrown toenails, impetigo, athlete's foot, warts, contact dermatitis, and nodules or abnormalities and for overall skin health.

Musculoskeletal Examination

Assess patients for any pain on palpation (POP) of the leg foot and ankle. Clinicians should evaluate patients for brachymetatarsia, polydactyly, clinodactyly, hammertoes, and abnormal growths. Muscle strength should be assessed to all plantarflexors, dorsiflexors, inverters, and everters of the foot.

A comprehensive pediatric examination is crucial for accurate diagnosis and subsequent treatment. The special needs of pediatric patients must be taken into account as well as the need to communicate findings with parents or caregivers to the children while making children feel comfortable and included in the discussion.

REFERENCES

1. Valmassy RL. Clinical biomechanics of the lower extremities. St Louis (MO): Mosby; 1996. p. 149 Chapter 7, Gait evaluation in clinical biomechanics, by C.C. Southerland, Jr.

2. Heath CH, Staheli LT. Normal limits of knee angle in white children–genu varum and genu valgum. J Pediatr Orthop 1993;13(2):259–62.
3. Salenius P, Vankka E. The development of the tibiofemoral angle in children. J Bone Joint Surg Am 1975;57(2):259–61.
4. Kling TF Jr, Hensinger RN. Angular and torsional deformities of the lower limbs in children. Clin Orthop Relat Res 1983;(176):136–47.
5. Cass A, Canasta C. A review of tarsal coalition and pes planovalgus: clinical examination, diagnostic imaging, and surgical planning. J Foot Ankle Surg 2010;49: 274–93.
6. Singh D. Nils Sifverskiold (1888-1957) and gastrocnemius contracture. J Foot Ankle Surg 2013;19(2):135–8.
7. Sobel E, Levitz SJ, Caselli MA, et al. Reevaluation of the relaxed calcaneal stance position. Reliability and normal values in children and adults. J Am Podiatr Med Assoc 1999;89(5):258–64.
8. Sankar WN, Weiss J, Skaggs DL. Orthopaedic conditions in the newborn. J Am Acad Orthop Surg 2009;17(2):112–22.
9. Barlow TG. Early diagnosis and treatment of congenital dislocation of the hip. J Bone Joint Surg Br 1962;44:292–301.
10. Ortolani M. Congenital hip dysplasia in the light of early and very early diagnosis. Clin Orthop Relat Res 1976;(119):6–10.
11. Manske R, Prohaska D. Physical examination and imaging of the acute multiple ligament knee injury. N Am J Sports Phys Ther 2008;3(4):191–7.
12. Walker HK. Clinical methods: the history, physical, and laboratory examinations. 3rd edition. Boston: Butterworths; 1990.
13. Agnew P. McGlamry comprehensive textbook of foot and ankle surgery chapter 73 metatarsus adductus and allied disorders. 4th edition (1). Philadelphia: Wolters Kluwer Health Lippincott Williams and Wilkins; 2013. p. 1056–60.
14. Pokrassa M. McGlamry comprehensive textbook of foot and ankle surgery chapter 29 clubfoot. 3rd edition (1). Philadelphia: Wolters Kluwer Health Lippincott Williams and Wilkins; 2001. p. 1060–88.
15. Dimeglio A, Bensahel H, Souchet P, et al. Classification of clubfoot. J Pediatr Orthop B 1995;4:129–36.
16. Mathias R. Parani method of staging clubfeet. 2007. Photograph. GlobalClubfoot. orgWeb. 6 Jul 2013. Available at: http://globalclubfoot.org/ponseti/pirani-scoring/. Accessed July 6, 2013.
17. Senes FM, Campus R, Becchetti F, et al. Sciatic nerve injection palsy in the child: early microsurgical treatment and long-term results. Microsurgery 2009;29(6): 443–8.
18. Dyer PJ, Davis N. The role of the Pirani scoring system in the management of club foot by the Ponseti method. J Bone Joint Surg Br 2006;88:1082–4.
19. Downey M, Alison D. McGlamry comprehensive textbook of foot and ankle surgery chapter 45 tarsal coalition. 4th edition (1). Philadelphia: Wolters Kluwer Health Lippincott Williams and Wilkins; 2013. p. 600–37.
20. Green D, Williams M. McGlamry comprehensive textbook of foot and ankle surgery chapter 48 arthroereisis. 4th edition (1). Philadelphia: Wolters Kluwer Health Lippincott Williams and Wilkins; 2013. p. 677–91.
21. Smith G. McGlamry comprehensive textbook of foot and ankle surgery chapter 25 cavus foot. 3rd edition (1). Philadelphia: Wolters Kluwer Health Lippincott Williams and Wilkins; 2001. p. 855–90.
22. Whitney AK, Green Dr. Pseudoequinus. 1 Am Podiatry Assoc 1982;72:365–71.

23. Chandrasekhar A. Meddean.luc.edu. Loyola University Medical Education Network. N.p., 28 Mar 2006. Web. 6 Jul 2013. Available at: http://www.meddean.luc.edu/lumen/meded/medicine/pulmonar/pd/contents.htm.

24. Niechwiej-Szwedo E, González E, Bega S, et al. "Proprioceptive role for palisade endings in extraocular muscles: evidence from the Jendrassik Maneuver". Vision Res 2006;46(14):2268–79. http://dx.doi.org/10.1016/j.visres.2005.12.006.

25. Lowe W. The Trendelenburg Sign. 2011. Photograph. MassageToday.comWeb. 6 Jul 2013. Available at: http://www.massagetoday.com/mpacms/mt/article.php?id=14379.

26. Mosca V. Clubfoot. 2013. Photograph. Seattle Children's Hospital Web. 6 Jul 2013. Available at: http://www.seattlechildrens.org/medical-conditions/bone-joint-muscle-conditions/clubfoot/.

27. Kumar SP, Ramasurbramanian D. The Babinski sign-a reappraisal. Neurol India 2000;48:314.

28. McGlamry DE, Jimenez AL, Green DR. McGlamry comprehensive textbook of foot and ankle surgery chapter 9 lesser ray deformities. 3rd edition (1). Philadelphia: Wolters Kluwer Health Lippincott Williams and Wilkins; 2001. p. 280–343.

Pediatric Forefoot Pathology

Ramy Fahim, DPM[a,c], Zachary Thomas, DPM[b],
Lawrence A. DiDomenico, DPM, FACFAS[a,c],*

KEYWORDS

- Pediatric forefoot • Polydactyly • Macrodactyly

KEY POINTS

- The management of pediatric pedal deformities of any kind requires extreme vigilance.
- The pediatric bone has unique characteristics that warrant special consideration.
- Many times, at initial presentation, the only complaint of pain comes from the child's parent. A careful physical examination and history-taking can help sort through the decision tree.
- Approach with a vision of how ones intervention will affect the child later as he/she reaches skeletal maturity.

INTRODUCTION

Surgical management of the pediatric forefoot often brings challenges to the foot and ankle surgeon. It requires a thorough understanding of the pathologic abnormality and underlying causes involved, which include the contributing genetic conditions. Albeit most of the deformities carry a rare level of incidence, they do however have a significant level of psychological component and stress on the pediatric patient. The goals of managing those pathologic abnormalities are ultimately to improve function while achieving a cosmetically acceptable outcome. In this article the common forefoot pathologic abnormalities in the pediatric population are reviewed with an added focus toward management of forefoot trauma in that patient group.

POLYDACTYLY

Polydactyly is a common congenital condition involving the hands and feet. It is characterized by the presence of one ore more supernumerary digits, and in some cases metatarsal/metacarpal bones (**Fig. 1**). Involvement in the hand is typically twice as often as in the foot.[1] The condition is equally frequent among male and female patients with bilateral involvement seen in 25% to 50% of the patients.[1,2] In a study of 120,000 live births, Frazier found an incidence of 1.7/1000 births.[3,4]

[a] Ankle and Foot Care Centers/Kent State University College of Podiatric Medicine, 6000 Rockside Woods Boulevard Independence, OH 44131, USA; [b] Heritage Medical Center, Beaver, PA; [c] St. Elizabeth Hospital, 8175 Market Street, Youngstown, Ohio 44512, USA
* Corresponding author.
E-mail address: ld5353@aol.com

Clin Podiatr Med Surg 30 (2013) 479–490
http://dx.doi.org/10.1016/j.cpm.2013.07.007
0891-8422/13/$ – see front matter © 2013 Elsevier Inc. All rights reserved.
podiatric.theclinics.com

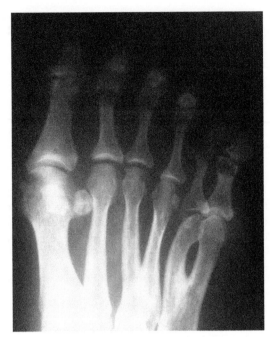

Fig. 1. Supernumerary digits and metatarsals of the right foot.

The pattern of inheritance and exact cause of polydactyly are not fully understood. Appoximately 15% of patients with polydactyly of the feet have an associated anomaly.[2] In addition, the condition is seen with autosomal-recessively inherited syndromes, such as Pallister-Hall, Lawrence-Moon-Bardet-Biedl, Ellis-Van Creveld, and various trisomies. A family history of polydactyly has also been reported in 10% to 30% of the subjects.[2,4]

Classification

Swanson in 1976[5] classified congenital limb malformations. The main categories included failure of formation of parts, failure of differentiation of parts, duplication, overgrowth (gigantism), undergrowth (hypoplasia), congenital constriction band syndrome, and generalized skeletal abnormalities.

Temtamy and McKusick classified polydactyly by determining whether the presentation was isolated or part of a syndrome. Within those categories, further subclassification is based on the anatomic location of the duplicated digits as either preaxial or postaxial. Preaxial refers to the tibial side of a line bisecting the second ray, whereas postaxial refers to the fibular sides. Postaxial polydactyly are subdivided into types A and B. Type A digits are fully developed with articulating skeletal structures, whereas type B are rudimentary digits. Postaxial type A polydactyly is the more common pattern.[6]

Venn-Watson[4] provided another classification based on the morphology of the corresponding metatarsal. The patterns from least differentiated to most differentiated were as follows: soft tissue duplication, wide metatarsal head, T-metatarsal, Y-metatarsal, and complete duplication.

Watanabe and colleagues[2] classified polydactyly by the type of ray involvement and level of duplication. The anatomic pattern types in medial-ray polydactyly are tarsal, metatarsal, proximal, and distal phalangeal. Central-ray types are metatarsal, proximal, middle, and distal phalangeal. Lateral-ray are subdivided into medial and lateral supernumerary toes.

Treatment

Surgical management of infants can often be addressed by early suture ligation or surgical excision.[7] General principles recommend saving the digit that is the most developed, has the most normal or anatomic MTP articulation, is most cosmetically acceptable, and is the one that will give the best contour to the foot.

Management of preaxial polydactyly is more complex with less optimum long-term results. Typically, the most medial digit is excised and additional tendon lengthening procedures, osteotomies, or other first ray soft tissue procedures may be used. Temporary pin fixation may be required to allow for soft tissue healing. However, complications of recurrent hallux varus and splaying of the first metatarsal are possible outcomes.

Postaxial polydactyly management has better and more predictable long-term results.[4,5] In most cases, the lateral-most digit is excised, usually through a racquet-type incisional approach. In addition, a block-metatarsal or wide-metatarsal head should be narrowed to a standard size to stabilize the joint. In the cases of T-shaped or Y-shaped metatarsals, the extra bone is typically resected to create a more standard metatarsal. Furthermore, in the cases of duplicated metatarsals, the entire ray should be removed. The transverse intermetatarsal ligament is also typically repaired in those cases to prevent splaying of the foot.

Central ray duplication has a more rare presentation but typically supernumerary central digits can be excised through a racquet-shaped incision with a dorsal arm. Similar to postaxial polydactyly in the cases of metatarsal duplication, the entire ray should be resected and a primary intermetatarsal ligament repair should be performed to prevent splaying.

MACRODACTYLY

Macrodactyly is considered a rare congenital deformity characterized by an increase in size of osseous and soft tissue structures of one or more digits.[8] Unilateral presentation of digits is the most common presentation and is typically seen with the first, second, and third toes. In addition, soft tissue overgrowth is also associated at the distal plantar aspect of the involved digit.[9] Although presentation in the foot is less common than in the hand, the deformity is more progressive.[10]

Although macrodactyly frequently occurs as an isolated congenital defect, literature supports association with neurofibromatosis-1, Klippel-Trenaunay-Parkes-Weber syndrome, hemihypertrophy, hemangiomatosis, arteriovenous fistula, lymphangiomatosis, and congenital lipofibromatosis.

The goals of surgical management of macrodactyly include achieving a plantigrade foot similar in width and length to the contralateral side. Treatment options include amputation, epiphyseal plate arrest, and different debulking procedures of the soft tissues. Potential complications include but are not limited to wound dehiscence, prolonged edema, and sensory disturbances.[11,12]

SYNDACTYLY

Syndactyly and polysyndactyly of the digits are common congenital deformities of the foot (**Fig. 2**). Unlike the hand, syndactyly is typically a cosmetic problem without any functional impairment. Thus, the treatment goals are indicated for cosmetic, psychological, and practical reasons.[13,14]

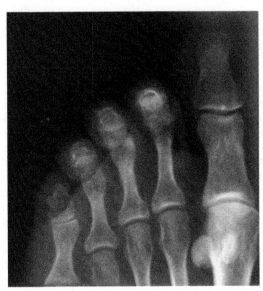

Fig. 2. Polysydactly of the lesser digits. Note the webbing between digits 2, 3, 4, and 5.

Classification

Davis and German[14] classified syndactyly into 4 main categories: (1) incomplete, the skin webbing between the 2 digits does not extend into the distal aspect of the digit; (2) complete, the skin webbing extends to the most distal aspect of the digits; (3) simple, no phalangeal involvement; and (4) complex, phalangeal bones are abnormal.

A well-accepted technique in the surgical management of syndactyly is the use of a dorsal rectangular flap and full-thickness skin grafts to provide additional skin cover, especially at the base of the digits. However, complications of donor site morbidity, hypertrophic scarring, web creep, pigmentation problems, contractures, and hair growth are possible. Other methods for surgical repair include the use of a xenograft for tissue coverage and various plastic surgical techniques, such as the V-flap or rectangular flap.[15]

BRACHYMETATARSIA

Brachymetatarsia was described by Kite as shortening of one or more metatarsals because of a premature fusion of the epiphyseal line at the distal end of the metatarsal (**Fig. 3**).[16] The causes range from traumatic, iatrogenic, and systemic to disorders that include pseudohypoparathyroidism, Turner syndrome, Albright hereditary osteodystrophy, and Down syndrome.[17,18] Females are affected by a 25:1 ratio and typically the fourth metatarsal has the highest rate of incidence.

Surgical correction is used to alleviate pain, establish acceptable cosmesis to the foot, and restore functional metatarsal parabola. Those include soft tissue correction such as the Kelekian syndactylization of lesser toes 4 and 5, use of joint spacers, bone-grafting techniques, and the Ilizarov method of callus distraction.[19]

METATARSAL FRACTURES

Fractures of the metatarsals in children can present several treatment dilemmas. Many practitioners abide by the "if the bones are in the same room they will heal" philosophy

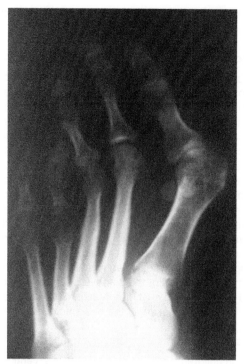

Fig. 3. Skeletal mature pediatric patient with a brachymetatarsal of the fourth metatarsal.

and others take a more aggressive stance. They also comprise most fractures seen by foot and ankle providers in children. In a study performed by The Cincinnati Children's Hospital they found that metatarsal fractures comprise 90% of all skeletal trauma in the foot in children with the fifth metatarsal being the most common of the 5 metatarsal bones to be acutely fractured and the second metatarsal being the most common bone subjected to stress fractures. A typical history of a child with a metatarsal stress fracture is that of a recent increase in activity or change of shoe or cleat. Radiographs are only diagnostic of about half the stress fractures seen in children so high suspicion is needed to diagnose an occult fracture. Magnetic resonance imaging may be used if suspicion is high. These injuries respond to immobilization in a cast for 3 to 6 weeks (Crawford AH, unpublished data, 1991).

Metatarsal Neck Fractures

Although metatarsal neck fractures are rare injuries, if there is no cartilaginous or epiphyseal involvement, most authors recommend a below-knee cast for 3 weeks. If surgical intervention is necessary, smooth K-wires are to be used to prevent physeal arrest or the development of growth aberrations.[20]

Metatarsal Shaft Fractures

These fractures occur usually from direct trauma. Transverse plane deviation is well tolerated; however, sagittal plane mal alignment can result in abnormal weight distribution and future metatarsalgia, stress syndromes, and digital deformities.[20] When casting with or without closed reduction can be performed, it is indicated otherwise, open reduction, internal fixation with internal fixation that does not violate the physis generates good results.

Metatarsal Base Fractures

Metatarsal base fractures rarely cause long-term problems except for the first metatarsal due to the proximal location of its epiphysis. These fractures are referred to as "buckle base" fractures owing to their tendency to buckle at the proximal epiphysis. If there is no displacement of the physis, these fractures heal uneventfully with short leg casting.[20] Fractures of the base of the fifth metatarsal become more common as children reach the age of playing competitive sports, namely sports that require repetitive jumping. Avulsion fractures of the fifth metatarsal base must be differentiated from a painful secondary ossification center or os vesalianum. Riccardi and colleagues[21] found that 47% of painful ossification centers of the fifth metatarsal base were misdiagnosed as fractures. Lawrence[22] expounded on the Stewart classification system to reflect pediatric injuries. The system is separated into 6 categories: (1) open growth plate apophyseal avulsions; (2) open growth plate apophyseal stress fractures (Iselin disease); (3) closed or closing growth plate tuberosity avulsion fractures; (4) Jones-type fractures through the metaphyseal–diaphyseal watershed area; (5) acute diaphyseal fractures; (6) stress fractures of the diaphysis. These fractures respond well to conservative care in a below-knee cast. If nonunion occurs, removal of the fragment may be needed but is rarely necessary in the pediatric population.

Phalangeal Fractures

Phalangeal fractures in children rarely warrant surgical intervention. Van Vliet-Koppert and colleagues[23] found that 95% of digital fractures were minimally or nondisplaced. In the review performed by Cincinnati Children's Hospital, it was found that the proximal phalanges were the most commonly fractured digital bone followed by the middle and distal (Crawford AH, unpublished data, 1991). Treatment consists of buddy splitting with a stiff-soled shoe. Displacement of the first proximal phalangeal base may warrant a closer look because of the propensity for the development of hallux limitus later in skeletal maturity. Open fractures in these spaces should be treated as any other stage 1 open fracture with irrigation and debridement; if the insult occurs around the nail complex, removal of the nail is warranted. These wounds are often closed primarily.[24]

Iselin's Disease

Overview

Traction epiphysitis of the base of the fifth metatarsal was originally described by Iselin in 1912. He noted this condition arose during adolescence. Iselin's disease is one of several osteochondroses found in the foot. Anatomically, the osteochondroses are categorized as articular, nonarticular, or physeal. This secondary center of ossification appears at about 10 years of age in girls and 12 years of age in boys.[25] This secondary ossification center can be seen well on medial oblique radiographs of the foot but is masked by the anterior-posterior and lateral projections.[26] The anatomic area in which Iselin's disease arises is unique in that the base of the fifth metatarsal fills all anatomic criteria for nonarticular osteochondrosis, being (1) the site of tendon attachment; (2) the site of ligamentous attachment; and (3) the site of impact.[25–27] Clinical diagnosis can be made with a typical history of pain on weight-bearing, participation in sports that require running, cutting, and jumping. The traction results from the pull of the peroneus brevis while the foot is inverted. Oftentimes edema can be noted around the base of the fifth metatarsal. Radiograph findings show fragmentation of the epiphysis and TC-99m bone scans will show increased uptake around the apophysis.

Treatment

Treatment consists of relative rest, icing, and anti-inflammatory medication. If no resolution of symptoms is noted with these modalities, the next stage in the treatment ladder is immobilization in a cast or CAM walker in the acute stages. A surgical shoe is not an ideal treatment because it cannot control the movement of the peroneus brevis muscle-tendinous unit. This condition has been noted to resolve spontaneously with the cessation of skeletal growth but nonunion has been noted.[26,28] Failure to recognize this diagnosis can cause long-term pain into adulthood. Differentiating a chronic or acute-on-chronic Iselin's disease from an avulsion fracture or stress fracture requires a thorough history because treatment likely will differ. Proximal stress fractures occur in diaphyseal bone, which is a key anatomic difference; however, Jones fractures have the potential to occur closer to the physis given their metaphyseal-diaphyseal location. Treatment of a base avulsion would be casting; however, if a nonunion has occurred that has been aggravated later in life, removal of the fragment would be the treatment of choice.[26] Differentiating chronic Iselin's nonunion versus a painful of vesalianum is not as critical in that the treatments are similar.

Freiberg Disease

Overview

Osteochondrosis of one or more metatarsal heads was originally described by Freiberg in 1914. It is more common in female teenagers than male teenagers and the second metatarsal head is most commonly affected, followed by the third metatarsal head.[27] Repetitive microtrauma is the most accepted etiologic theory despite Freiberg's original theory of a single traumatic event being the causative factor. It was a common misconception that increased plantar pressure from an elongated second metatarsal was the cause of this transient osteonecrosis; however, Gauthier and Elbaz[29] in their study found no correlation between second metatarsal length and risk of osteonecrosis. Some authors think that a genetic predisposition is present in the development of this osteonecrosis. Blitz and Yu[30] published a case report of identical twins developing Freiberg infarction in which they used this data to elucidate a genetic root cause. Radiographs typically show flattening of the involved metatarsal head with sclerosis, fragmentation, and early joint space widening[29] and over time the joint will show typical signs of arthrosis. Magnetic resonance imaging is reserved for atypical radiographic presentations or to differentiate stress fracture or osteomyelitis. Usually, depending on the level of necrosis, the involved metatarsal will show low signal intensity on both T1 and T2 sequence.[31]

Treatment

Acute therapy involves a period of non-weight-bearing with icing and anti-inflammatory medications. If this condition becomes chronic, conservative measures include offloading with a custom-molded orthoses that offload the metatarsal heads. Surgical interventions include chilectomy and joint remodeling, dorsiflexory closing wedge osteotomy of the involved metatarsal head that brings unaffected cartilage into the joint space, total joint arthroplasty, metatarsal head resection, and osteochondral autograft transfer system (OATS) transplant. Arthrodiastasis has also recently been described to treat chondrocyte damage either alone or as an adjunct. DeVries and colleagues[32] described a surgical technique in which they combined osteochondral autograft transfer system (OATS) transfer of the involved metatarsal head from the femoral distal lateral condyle, which was augmented with mini-rail external fixation for

6 weeks. Interpositional arthroplasty using the extensor digitorum longus tendon has also been described for surgeons wary of total joint arthroplasty.[33]

INSERT SMILIE CLASSIFICATION
Longitudinal Epiphyseal Bracket

Overview
Longitudinal epiphyseal bracket (LEB) is a congenital anomaly affecting the tubular bones of the hand and foot in which the proximal epiphysis is L-shaped or C-shaped and runs along the medial border of the bone; this results in the formation of a short, trapezoidal bone caused by the bone growing in more of a mediolateral direction instead of longitudinally.[34,35] The great toe is affected in 11% of all cases of LEB, or "Delta Phalanx," as is it was originally described.[36] Conditions associated with LEBs include the following: hallux varus, polydactaly, Rubenstein-Taybi, diastrophic dwarphism, Apert syndrome, syndactyly, ulnar and cleft hands, and tibial hemimelia.[35,37] Radiographically, the bracket can be visualized from 2 to 11 years of age.

Treatment
The stalwart of treatment of this condition is surgical resection of the bracket. Timing of surgical intervention is ideally during the first year of life to allow the affected bone to experience normal longitudinal growth. Further reasoning for resection of the bracket early in life is because there is still no bone overgrowing the bracket. Once ossification occurs over the bracket, bone must be resected to reach it, which increases the chance of disturbing the longitudinal physis. Adjunctive procedures include opening wedge osteotomy, which may be performed as part of the original surgery or as a staged procedure. There is also a role for callus distraction with external fixation.[38] Also, tendon lengthening may be needed as the tendinous unit may have modeled around the shortened bone.

JUVENILE HAV
Overview

Ninety percent of hallux valgus is hereditary (**Fig. 4**).[39] Pediatric hallux valgus presents several unique treatment dilemmas. Many times the child will present, pre-empted by a worried parent, with no pain whatsoever. Other times, the child may present with a hallux valgus deformity as part of a larger scale limb length discrepancy, metatarsus adductus, skewfoot, or painful flatfoot deformity that sincerely limits activity. The physis of the first metatarsal is located proximal along the bone unlike the other 4 metatarsals. Occasionally, a pseudoepiphysis will appear at the distal metaphyseal-epiphyseal junction. In male children, the proximal physis can appear from age 5 months to as late as 2.3 years in and from birth to 2 years in female children and closes anywhere from 13 to 22 years of age. The first step in any treatment algorithm for juvenile HAV should be a thorough radiographic, neuromuscular, and biomechanical examination.[40] McCluney and Tinley found significant radiologic parameters for differentiating juvenile HAV from a normal foot to be a 15 degree or more metatarsus primus adductus angle and a positively met protrusion index.[41] A pediatric bunion will invariably have some component of hypermobility, especially when dealing with pediatric hypermobile flatfoot. A Silfverskiold test should be performed to determine the role of equinus in driving the deformity.

Treatment

The first step in the treatment of juvenile patients is to support the foot with orthoses. In some cases, a deep-seated heel cup may be used to control a flexible flatfoot. A heel

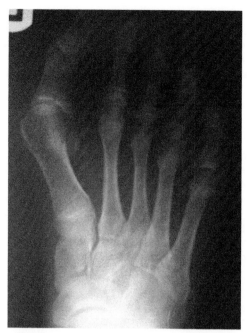

Fig. 4. An anterior-posterior radiograph demonstrating a significant hallux abducto valgus deformity in a pediatric patient.

lift should be placed on the contralateral limb to stop abnormal subtalar joint pronation of the affected side if a limb length difference is measured. If there is a larger scale abnormality driving the hallux valgus such as a rigid flatfoot caused by tarsal coalition, this condition will dictate treatment. Watchful waiting is also an acceptable treatment algorithm if the child is in no pain and still has many formative years ahead.[40] In this philosophy, the surgeon waits until the physis is near closure at the time of adolescence and at that time a modified Lapidus is performed. In the adolescent population, a hallux valgus deformity with an associated hypermobile first ray can present a treatment challenge. This mechanical abnormality, when presenting in adults, can be corrected with predictability using a modified lapidus bunionectomy.[42,43] In pediatric patients, however, this procedure has great potential to violate the proximal physis of the first metatarsal in patients who are not near skeletal maturity; thus, there is a certain popularity of the long-arm chevron osteotomy in this patient population that still has growth potential from the proximal physis. Some surgeons in the past have opted for soft tissue rebalancing procedures in this population; however, these procedures are fraught with recurrence.[44] Other options include an oblique closing base wedge osteotomy placed distal to the physis. This osteotomy does involve diaphyseal bone; however, the pediatric bone potential for healing should be considered. Medial cuneiform opening wedge osteotomy, originally described by Cotton in 1935, has also been used in the pediatric population as a procedure to maintain length of the first ray, although this procedure should not be performed until the age of 6 when the medial column has fully ossified.[45] Some surgeons choose to use the proximal physis to their advantage with epiphysiodesis procedures in an attempt to correct the angle of growth before most longitudinal growth occurs in the first metatarsal; however, this is a challenging surgical option and the potential for undercorrection or overcorrection is high and it must be performed on the younger pediatric population for any success to be achieved. Achilles tendon lengthening or gastrocnemius recession should always be considered an adjunctive procedure if equinus contracture is present; if this driving force is not corrected, recurrence will inevitably occur because of a tight heel cord causing abnormal subtalar joint pronation and unlocking of the transverse tarsal joint.

DISCUSSION

The management of pediatric pedal deformities of any kind requires extreme vigilance. The pediatric foot should not be considered a miniature adult foot. The pediatric bone has unique characteristics that warrant special consideration. Many times, at initial presentation, the only complaint of pain comes from the child's parent. A careful physical examination and history-taking can help sort through the decision tree. In this article, an overview of the pathologic pediatric digits and metatarsals has been given as well as treatment algorithms for several digital and metatarsal derangements. Any deformity in children should be approached with a vision of how one's intervention will affect the child later as he/she reaches skeletal maturity.

REFERENCES

1. Masada K, Tsuyuguchi Y, Kawabata H, et al. Treatment of preaxial polydactyly of the foot. Plast Reconstr Surg 1987;79:251–8.
2. Watanabe H, Fujita S, Oka I. Polydactyly of the foot: an analysis of 265 cases and a morphological classificaion. Plast Reconstr Surg 1992;89:856–77.
3. Frazier TM. A note on race-specific congenital malformation rates. Amer J Obstet Gynec 1960;80:184–5.
4. Venn-Watson EA. Problems in polydactyly of the foot. Orthop Clin North Am 1976; 7:909–27.
5. Swanson AB. A classification for congenital limb malformations. J Hand Surg 1976;1:8–22.
6. Temtamy SA, McKusick VA. Synopsis of hand malformations with particular emphasis on genetic factors. Birth Defects 1969;5:125–84.
7. Ruby L, Goldberg M. Syndactyly and polydactyly. Orthop Clin North Am 1976;7: 361–74.
8. Barsky AJ. Macrodactyly. J Bone Joint Surg Am 1967;49:1255–65.
9. DeValentine S, Scurran BL, Turek D, et al. Macrodactyly of the lower extremity: a review with two case reports. J Am Podiatry Assoc 1981;71:175–80.
10. Dennyson WG, Bear JN, Bhoola KD. Macrodactyly in the foot. J Bone Joint Surg Br 1977;59:355–9.
11. De Greef A, Pretorius LK. Macrodactyly: a review with a case report. S Afr Med J 1983;63:939–41.
12. Tsuge K. Treatment of macrodactyly. Plast Reconstr Surg 1967;3:590–9.
13. Alder J, Gentless J, Springer K, et al. Concomitant syndactyly and polydactyly in a pediatric foot. J Foot Ankle Surg 1997;36(2):151–4.
14. Davis JS, German WJ. Syndactylism (coherence of fingers and toes). Arch Surg 1930;21:32–75.
15. Bouchard JL. Congenital deformities of the foot, ch.18. In: Comprehensive textbook of foot surgery, vol. 1. American Medical Association. p. 588–91.
16. Kite JH. The club foot. New York: Grune and Stratton; 1964. p. 156.
17. Handelman RB, Perlman MD, Coleman WB. Brachymetatarsia: a review of the literature and case report. J Am Podiatr Med Assoc 1986;76:413–6.

18. Ferrandez L, Yubero J, Usabiaga J, et al. Congenital brachymetatarsia: three cases. Foot Ankle 1993;14:529–33.
19. Bartolomei FJ. Sugical correction of brachymetatarsia. J Am Podiatr Med Assoc 1990;80:76–82.
20. Green NE, Swiontkowski MF. Skeletal trauma in children. 4th edition. MO: Elsevier; 2008.
21. Riccardi G, Riccardi D, Marcarelli M, et al. Extremely proximal fractures of the fifth metatarsal in the developmental age. Foot Ankle Int 2011;32(5):S526–32.
22. Lawrence SJ. Technique tip: local bone grafting technique for Jones fracture management with intramedullary screw fixation. Foot Ankle 2004;25:920–1.
23. Van Vliet-Koppert ST, Cakir H, Van Lieshout EM, et al. Demographics and functional outcome of toe fractures. J Foot Ankle Surg 2011;50(3):307–10.
24. Okike K, Bhattacharyya T. Trends in the management of open fractures. A critical analysis. J Bone Joint Surg Am 2006;88:2739–48.
25. Canale ST, Beaty JH. Campbell's operative orthopaedics. 11th edition. MO: Mosby, An Imprint of Elsevier; 2007.
26. Ralph BG, Barrett J, Kenyhercz C, et al. Iselin's disease: a case presentation of nonunion and review of the differential diagnosis. Journal of Foot and Ankle Surgery 1999 Nov-Dec;38(6):409–16.
27. DeLee JC. DeLee and Drez's orthopaedic sports medicine. 3rd edition. MO: Saunders, An Imprint of Elsevier; 2009.
28. Schwartz B, Jay RM, Schoenhaus HD. Apophysitis of the fifth metatarsal base. Iselin's disease. J Foot Ankle Surg 1999;38(6):409–16.
29. Gauthier G, Elbaz R. Freiberg's infraction: a subchondral bone fatigue fracture. A new surgical treatment. Clin Orthop Relat Res 1979;(142):93–5.
30. Blitz NM, Yu JH. Freiberg's infraction in identical twins: a case report. J Foot Ankle Surg 2005;44(3):218–21.
31. Patel CV. The foot and ankle: MR imaging of uniquely pediatric disorders. Magn Reson Imaging Clin N Am 2009;17:539–47, vii.
32. DeVries JG, Amiot RA, Cummings P, et al. Freiberg's infraction of the second metatarsal treated with autologous osteochondral transplantation and external fixation. J Foot Ankle Surg 2008;47(6):565–70.
33. El-Tayeby H. Freiberg's infraction: a new surgical procedure. J Foot Ankle Surg 1998;37(1):23–7.
34. Kucukkaya M, Mehmet Y, Kuzgun T. Correcting and lengthening of metatarsal deformity with circular fixator by distraction osteotomy: a case of longitudinal epiphyseal bracket. J Am Podiatr Med Assoc 1991;81(3):128–30.
35. Schreck MA. Pediatric longitudinal epiphyseal bracket: review and case presentation. J Foot Ankle Surg 2006;45(5):342–5.
36. Jones GB. Delta phalanx. J Bone Joint Surg Br 1964;46:226–8.
37. Mubarak SJ, O'Brien TJ, Davids JR. Metatarsal epiphyseal bracket: treatment by central physiolysis. J Pediatr Orthop 1993;13(1):5–8.
38. Scott R, Kissel C, Miller A. Correction of longitudinal epiphyseal bracket disease with external fixation: a case report with 6-year follow-up period. J Foot Ankle Surg 2011;50:714–7.
39. Piqué-Vidal C, Solé MT, Antich J. Hallux valgus inheritance: pedigree research in 350 patients with bunion deformity. J Foot Ankle Surg 2007;46(3):149–54.
40. Harris EJ, Vanore JV, Thomas JL, et al, Clinical Practice Guideline Pediatric Flatfoot Panel of the American College of Foot and Ankle Surgeons. Diagnosis and treatment of pediatric flatfoot. J Foot Ankle Surg 2004;43(6):341–73.

41. McCluney JG, Tinley P. Radiographic measurements of patients with juvenile hallux valgus comparedwith age-matched controls: a cohort investigation. J Foot Ankle Surg 2006;45(3):161–7.
42. Lagaay PM, Hamilton GA, Ford LA, et al. Rates of revision surgery using chevron-austin osteotomy, lapidus arthrodesis, and closing base wedge osteotomy for correction of hallux valgus deformity. J Foot Ankle Surg 2008;47(4):267–72.
43. Patel S, Ford LA, Etcheverry J, et al. Modified lapidus arthrodesis: rate of nonunion in 227 cases. J Foot Ankle Surg 2004;43(1):37–42.
44. Davids JR, McBrayer D, Blackhurst DW. Juvenile hallux valgus deformity: surgical management by lateral hemiepiphyseodesis of the great toe metatarsal. J Pediatr Orthop 2007;27(7):826–30.
45. Lynch FR. Applications of the opening wedge cuneiform osteotomy in the surgical repair of juvenile hallux abducto valgus. J Foot Ankle Surg 1995;34(2):103–23.

Pediatric First Ray Deformities

Patrick Agnew, DPM, FACFAS, FACFAP*

KEYWORDS

- Juvenile • Hallux valgus • Symptomatic • Surgery

KEY POINTS

- Pediatric first ray deformities may present in many ways similar to those effecting adults.
- Management of the patient and the deformity necessitates special consideration of timing, the patient's general health, techniques, and perhaps goals.
- Any simple broad brush approach to the care of these patients will certainly result in both undertreatment and overtreatment.
- Proper care is an ongoing process of appropriate management tailored to the patient's needs, deformities, and developmental age.
- Proper adherence to these recommendations can improve the patient's quality of life and result in a gratifying professional experience for the dedicated health care provider.

INTRODUCTION

According to Garrison Keeler, in "Lake Woebegone," Minnesota: "the women are strong, the men are good looking and all of the children are above average." However, not all children are alike, and children are not little adults (James V. Ganley, DPM, personal communication, 1986) (**Fig. 1**). Furthermore, not all bunions are alike. Is there a deformity at the interphalangeal joint? The metatarsal phalangeal joint? The metatarsal cuneiform joint? All of the metatarsals? The tarsometatarsal joints, any or all of the above. Is the child complaining? Are the deformities causing disability? Are they progressing?

Management decision making in this population is particularly challenging. Carefully evaluating the goals of the patient and their family is essential. The short-term and long-term objectives should be included. The durability of any treatment should be considered. Is a permanent result even a realistic expectation? The treating provider's medical legal exposure to the statute of limitations may extend until the child becomes an adult.

CAUSE

The cause of first ray deformities is probably multifactorial. Very rarely is an infant borne with hallux valgus (abnormally high hallux abductus angle). Even metatarsus

Eastern Virginia Medical School, c/o Coastal Podiatry 6477 College Park Square, Suite 108, Virginia Beach, Norfolk, VA 23464, USA
* 6477 College Park Square, Suite 108, Virginia Beach, VA 23464.
E-mail address: pagnw@aol.com

Clin Podiatr Med Surg 30 (2013) 491–501
http://dx.doi.org/10.1016/j.cpm.2013.07.005
0891-8422/13/$ – see front matter © 2013 Elsevier Inc. All rights reserved.

podiatric.theclinics.com

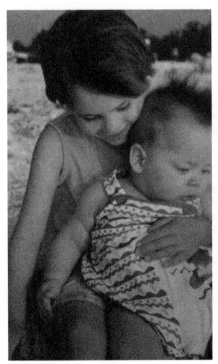

Fig. 1. Children are not little adults. Notice the head size to arm length differences between the infant and his 4-year-old sister.

adductus may be a deformity, possibly caused by interuterine forces, as opposed to a true malformation (a packaging defect vs a manufacturing defect). Similarly, hallux interphalangeal abnormalities are commonly inherited, but rarely identified congenitally. Exceptions such as delta phalanx are rare causes. Predisposition to acquired deformities of the first ray is not well researched, although interesting theories abound. In 1 theory,[1] overpronation of the hind foot causes a loss of mechanical advantage for the fibularis longus. This allows the first metatarsal to drift and adapt to a dorsiflexed position in weight bearing. Because the first metatarsal cuneiform joint supinates and pronates, the metatarsal also rotates in the frontal plane. It also drifts and adapts to a more medial position relative to the midline of the body. The hallux remains tethered to the rest of the foot by the intrinsic foot muscles and ligaments so the hallux abductus angle increases. Factors such as low muscle tone and loose ligaments may also contribute to overpronation of the foot.[2,3]

A casual examination of the family of a child with a first ray deformity usually reveals that something has been inherited (**Fig. 2**). Inappropriate footwear did not cause the deformity. Fossils have been found with first ray deformities in unshod prehistoric humanoids. In equatorial areas, there are many overpronating feet with a variety of first ray deformities (**Fig. 3**). So what was inherited? Familial hypermobility? Collagen disease? Neurologic disease? Muscle wasting disease? An effort to identify these potential contributing factors may help the provider to develop a prognosis. However, the bottom line is that whatever is wrong with the child's foot at birth (valgus tendency, varus tendency, equinus) will likely become worse, faster with any of the above comorbidities. That is essential heritable disease knowledge for the foot specialist in a nutshell.

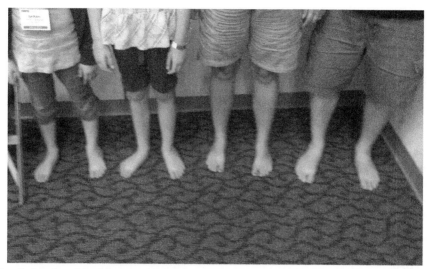

Fig. 2. Family with Ehlers-Danlos syndrome. Notice the presence of varying degrees of overpronation.

Rheumatic diseases are a rare contributor to pediatric first ray deformities, although some may severely exacerbate pediatric deformities when these diseases manifest later in life.

Congenital and childhood diseases may also be exacerbating factors. Spastic, flaccid, or athetotic cerebral palsy is caused by, usually static, incidents that affect the central nervous system before maturity. However, the manifestations in the foot may be relentlessly progressive. Whatever the foot was like at birth usually becomes progressively worse in these scenarios. Infectious diseases may directly alter the first ray by contiguous focus of course. Effects of infections (even remote in size and/or place) may stimulate autoimmune responses that may lead to progressive joint disruption anywhere, including the feet. An effort to identify these comorbidities is necessary out of concern for the patient's overall health. Referral to appropriate providers for care of these conditions may be necessary.

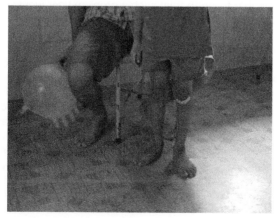

Fig. 3. Overpronation and digital deformities in an unshod or minimally shod family.

MANAGEMENT

Pediatric foot care is full of controversy. This is mostly because of a dearth of data. For really applicable data, a treatment and a control group would need to be watched for 20 years or more. Few investigators are active in research long enough. Few parents want their children in a control group. The data that are available are sometimes misinterpreted. With all due respect to the investigators, children inspire emotion. Jesus said: "As bad as you are, you know how to give good things to your children."[4] When opinions are discussed in pediatrics, they are often strongly defended.

My opinions (and these are only opinions) on methods of managing pediatric first ray deformities are presented in this article. Ideally, a protocol for primary care providers should be widely accepted. This would include early recognition of abnormalities and a focused patient and family history and physical examination. Telling a family that most children outgrow a problem when the mother has just had foot surgery and the grandmother is crippled may not impress the family. Evidence of the coexistence of lower extremity pathomechanics with lower extremity deformity is plentiful even though cause and effect correlations are lacking.[5]

INFANCY

Unfortunately, decisions are usually made based on the age at presentation. Infants may be presented with concerns about deformities of the first ray. Despite reliable and dedicated referring primary care providers, this author rarely sees these cases. Lesser digit, hind foot, and other lower extremity concerns are much more common in our experience. Incidence data and widely accepted treatment protocols are not available. Even highly discussed entities that may include first ray deformities remain controversial. Metatarsus adductus, for example, may involve some, all, or sometimes just the first metatarsal. This may not be clinically obvious and is difficult to discern even with imaging. Should this be treated (regardless of specific metatarsal involvement)? If so, how? When? That depends on whose philosophy you follow. Staheli and colleagues[6] believe that most infants outgrow many problems. Kite[7] believed that a day that a deformity is permitted to go untreated is a golden opportunity lost. Parents do not really care if most infants seem to outgrow a problem. They want to know if their infant will. No reliable method of predicting whether or not a given infant will outgrow metatarsus primus adductus, calcaneal valgus, or many other congenital abnormalities has been reported. No one who has ever spent any time around a toddler would argue that trying to treat such a problem later would be easier. Some correction, however, may be possible with relatively conservative methods until later in childhood.[8]

The author recommends an attempt to correct metatarsus adductus in infancy via casting, possibly followed by customizable shoe or splint maintenance. This is, however, a delicate procedure, "like molding wax."[6] It may be easier for the hind foot to pronate (normal motion) than for metatarsals or tarsals to remodel. Stabilizing the hind foot is therefore essential to avoid creating a new second deformity including overpronation (sometimes called skew foot or z foot). The first metatarsal phalangeal and interphalangeal areas must not be damaged with casting material to avoid creating hallux valgus and/or interphalangeal deformity. If deformities already exist at this level, cohesive elastic tape may be considered to try to remodel the involved bones. Remember that in infants "the soft tissues are hard, and the hard tissues are soft" (Richard Jay, DPM, 1984 lecture at the former Pennsylvania College of Podiatric Medicine). Ligaments may be more difficult to remodel than bones fortunately. Again, this may not be the case in patients with collagen disorders. Surgical treatment of these deformities is usually not recommended. Data on outcomes are rare and in some cases disappointing.[9] Periodic (at least annual) reevaluation is recommended.

Orthodigital devices lack supportive data and may be difficult to use as patients rapidly develop the ability to remove them. However, encouraging support by parents may result in compliance with use. Use while sleeping may be particularly acceptable and beneficial. Children spend most of their time sleeping and do most of their growing during that time, preferably in the right direction. Any risk of harm with such intervention seems negligible. Potential long-term benefit remains uncertain.

TODDLERS

From about 1 to 3 years of age, weight bearing may unmask abnormalities and stimulate presentation to a provider. Dynamic metatarsus adductus and/or hallux varus may be noticed. Overpronation, a likely risk factor for later development of first ray deformity, may still be difficult to recognize. The plantar fat pad may still be thick enough to mask the presence or absence of a plantar longitudinal foot arch.

Metatarsus adductus may still be corrected with casting or improved with splinting, although many toddlers may vehemently disagree. Surgical lengthening of the abductor hallucis tendon may be considered, although long-term results may be uncertain.[10] Overcorrection may conceivably cause hallux valgus (a much more common problem later in life than metatarsus adductus).

Exacerbating conditions such as ankle equinus must also be identified and treated. Failure to identify and resolve this leads to failure of orthotic or even invasive treatment of foot deformity. Night splinting may be tolerated and can influence corrected growth during the child's long sleep/growth daily. Invasive treatment may be considered if conservative treatment fails. Treatment of this component alone may even obviate invasive treatment of the presenting complaint of bunion pain by facilitating the use of orthotics and appropriate footwear. Invasive treatment of equinus is not without risks, however, including overcorrection, undercorrection, and neurovascular injury. The consequences of these types of complications may be permanent.

The influence of deformity on related structures such as toenails must also be considered. The toddler who keeps getting in-growing toenails or is developing onychodystrophy may have hallux valgus as a contributing comorbidity.

Soft tissue release of digital deformities may be cautiously considered. Severe deformity, especially with pain, may indicate that an attempt should be made. Again, long-term outcomes are uncertain, and special surgical risks such as growth plate damage exist.

The ability of the patient and parents to cooperate with postoperative care may be limited. Novel approaches with potential minimal postoperative care requirements may gain acceptance in the future. These may include botulism toxin injection of the adductor hallucis muscles and/or suture and button/anchor procedures to correct metatarsus primus adductus and/or hallux valgus.[11–13] These may conceivably permit remodeling of related joints and constructive redirection of growth.

PRESCHOOL AND KINDERGARTEN

Children in this age group have increasing societal demands to wear shoes. Protection of the feet from temperature extremes and trauma becomes necessary as the child ventures outside the home. Mature gate and foot structure will likely not be achieved yet. Biomechanical assessment may still not be reliable. Treating mild abnormalities such as apparent overpronation is controversial. Stigmatization may already be happening for children with an abnormal gait.

Concerns about the effects of treatment on the children's emotional development have been raised.[14] Controversy about this conclusion exists, however, because the different types of orthotics were not separated. Forest Gump may have been at greater risk of embarrassment than a 5-year-old soccer star who falls less often when wearing gait plates. The author advocates the use of neutral position foot orthoses, firm enough to control overpronation. This may slow or stop the development of foot deformities related to overpronation, including metatarsus primus adductus and hallux valgus.

In the rare cases of painful first ray deformities in this age group, options exist. An effort should be made to rule out comorbidities that may contribute to the deformity and symptoms. The causes of pain in this age group may even include psychosocial problems in the child's environment. Asking the parent(s) to consider this possibility and specific questions may reveal the potential pursuit of secondary gains by the child.

Four approaches to pain mitigation in this group may include: accommodation, analgesics, surgery, and monitored benign neglect (**Table 1**). Accommodation of the deformity may be accomplished with well-chosen or custom-made footwear. This may be easier at this age then later because the boney prominences are usually covered with baby fat. Essentially all analgesics carry some risks. Vital organ damage, drug interactions, blood dyscrasias, tolerance, addiction, and dependence are just some of the physical and psychological risks. Joint damage from interarticular medication and slight risk of infection limit their use. Inconsistent results, expense, inconvenience, limited access, and stigmatization may accompany physical modalities such as transcutaneous nerve stimulation. Topical compounded analgesics may hold some promise, but clear indications, potential side effects, and proper dosing are lacking. Quality control has recently become a grave concern with fungal infections occurring in many states from compounded injectables.

Table 1
Four approaches to mitigate symptoms related to hallux valgus and related deformities; equinus must be managed at any and all ages

	Age Group at Presentation			
Approach	Infancy	Toddlers	School Age	Adolescents
Accommodation	Footwear Orthodigital	Footwear	Footwear Orthodigital Orthotics	Footwear Orthodigital Orthotics
Analgesia	NSAIDs Topical	NSAIDs Topical	NSAIDs Topical Narcotic Physical modalities	NSAIDs Topical Narcotics Physical modalities
Surgery	Soft tissue balancing Osteotomies	Soft tissue balancing Stable osteotomies Bone anchors	Soft tissue balancing Osteotomies Bone anchors and suture Suture and buttons Epiphysiodesis	Soft tissue balancing Osteotomies Bone anchors suture Suture and buttons

Surgery is not commonly indicated in this age group. However, after a thorough workup to rule out the causes of symptoms other than the deformity and when conservative efforts have failed, surgical treatment may be considered. Parental consent must be obtained for all invasive procedures on minors. In children who have achieved an age of reason, the child's express consent should also be obtained. Special efforts to inform this age group may help to allay anxiety and increase the likelihood of satisfactory outcomes. Our children's hospital has classes available for patients and their families to prepare for upcoming procedures. Each age group typically has special concerns about invasive procedures.[15] This age group typically fears separation; and may begin to understand and fear pain and death. Parents may accompany our patients up to the operating suite and in rare cases enter the room in proper attire. Oral liquid or lollipop premedication is typically used, as well as mask induction.

Surgical options differ from those in adults. Soft tissue balancing, rarely indicated as a standalone procedure in adults (in the author's experience), may have a place in this age group. Lateral release of the metatarsal phalangeal joint, lateral sesamoid ligament, extensor hallucis brevis, and adductor hallucis conjoined tendons may correct hallux abductus deformity. Medial capsulorraphy of the surgeon's choice may also be effective to reinforce correction of that component of a deformity. The author sometimes uses a segment of the extensor hallucis brevis tendon to reinforce this repair as an onlay graft of the medial joint capsule (James V. Ganley, DPM, 1986, personal communication). After all, the medial joint capsule has already failed previously. Recently, we have been using small (2.7 mm) bone anchors, inserted percutaneously into the medial center of the metatarsal head and the proximal medial phalanx base. We then pass the swaged 2-0 polyester suture just superficial to the joint capsule and tie the strands together to correct the hallux abductus angle (**Fig. 4**). Long-term follow-up of this technique is not yet available, but early results in correcting relapses and treating patients with ligament laxity have been impressive. This is especially important in the latter group because of the potential for poor wound healing and difficult wound closure. No complications have been encountered yet. Caution to avoid the proximal phalanx growth plate is of course mandatory. The technique is performed

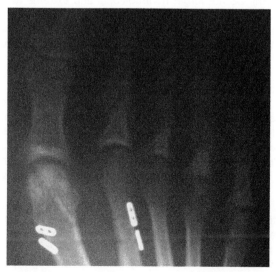

Fig. 4. 1.1 mm suture and button technique in a young adult.

with fluoroscopy. Therefore, the potential risks of radiation exposure to the patient must be weighed against the potential benefits of a stronger, durable repair with minimally invasive insertion. Extra protection of the patient's most vulnerable organs with shielding is necessary.

Correction of intermetatarsal angle presents special challenges and opportunities. Common osteotomy and arthrodesis procedures used in adults may have unpredictable results with continuing growth of the patient. Violation of growth plates may be an added risk with some procedures.

The risk of growth plate injury is also a potential opportunity. Partial epiphysiodesis may be an option now.[16] Again results may be difficult to predict with both undercorrection and overcorrection possible.

The natural flexibility of this age group may increase the likelihood of successful correction of the first intermetatarsal angle with suture and button techniques. Small (1.1 mm) drill hole methods are currently available to connect the first and second metatarsals. The special risk of these procedures, second metatarsal stress reactions, would seem less likely in young patients. The potential for remodeling of the first ray joints and bones is greater also, potentially producing more anatomic long-term results than osteotomies or arthrodesis.

SCHOOL-AGE CHILDREN

All 4 management options for this age group are essentially the same as those in the preschool age group. Exceptions include potentially better patient cooperation with treatments. This may include better compliance with noninvasive pain management strategies and perioperative behavior in surgical candidates. Treatment of any kind may become necessary in this age group as complaints may be more believable. Caution to rule out comorbidities and psychosocial causes of complaints must be exhaustive. Children in this age range are much more likely to adjust their reporting of the history of their present problem to fit the perceived expectations of their parents.

Organized and recreational activities may reveal symptoms related to previously unnoticed deformities. Request to examine specialized footwear (turf shoes, cleats, skates, and so forth). Do not forget nontraditional and extreme athletes. Shoes for skateboard riders may present an opportunity to help because they may accommodate orthotics well, or may do harm by being worn in inappropriate size by a fashion conscious child. Wetsuit booties are expensive for surfers, so wearing these beyond the time they have been outgrown may occur.

Some urgency to at least attempt maintenance/preventative intervention may exist at this age. Providers who tell the patient and the family that the child will outgrow the problem will not likely be accepted. The pathologically overpronated foot may no longer be dismissed as baby fat in the arch. Clinically obvious digital deformities do not spontaneously resolve. Progression is much more likely. Unaddressed first ray deformities may now possibly contribute to related problems such as avascular necrosis of nearby structures (eg, Freiberg disease). Antalgic gait caused by first ray deformity may conceivably contribute to otherwise seemingly remote conditions such as Kholer disease.

The use of orthotics to control overpronation is controversial. Some investigators have dismissed their usefulness with data showing that these efforts do not result in correction of overpronation.[17] That is not the goal of intervention. Optical glasses do not correct lens deformities either. They treat symptoms (headaches, and so forth) and prevent progression (academic failure). Similarly, although foot orthotics may not correct overpronation, they may prevent the progression of pronation-related deformities and their symptoms. Left alone, the entire weight-bearing skeleton un-doubtedly continues to adapt to the pathomechanics in the foundation, the feet. Admittedly, data to support this opinion are minimal. Claims to the contrary, however, are equally unfounded. A study to prove the theory that biomechanical control of the child's foot prevents the development or progression of deformities would require de-cades of follow-up and a control group whose parents are willing to decline potentially beneficial treatment. Matching cohorts would be extremely difficult in view of the different potential underlying causes of the foot problems, and the different stresses applied to the feet of the subjects. Double blinding seems impossible. So opinions persist. Data on the use of orthodigital devices are even less available.

Invasive treatment, although not commonly indicated, may be better accepted by children in this age group and their parents. They may also be more likely to evade complications. Children in this age group may be capable of cooperating with non–weight-bearing instructions, appropriate wound care, and activity restrictions. However, they may not want to. Their ingenuity in sabotaging the treating provider's efforts must not be underestimated.

Procedure selection is similar to that applied to preschool children but school-age children may have additional concerns. They may begin to fear scars and have often experienced some form of pain at this age, increasing their anxiety.

ADOLESCENTS

In our experience, the adolescent age group is the most common age group to self-present with complaints of pain and cosmetic concerns regarding first ray deformities. Rapid growth may suddenly increase first ray deformity. Overpronation may be exac-erbated by increasing body weight. Ankle equinus may appear or progress as bone growth outpaces muscle/tendon growth. Peer pressure to wear socially accepted footwear may lead to poor choices. Outgrowing shoes may exacerbate symptoms and may occur too fast for parents to realize.

Special attention to the goals of the patient is critical in adolescents. The desire to wear a particularly popular shoe may overwhelm reasonable concerns about potential complications of treatment. An honest history of symptoms may be difficult to obtain in the face of such a hidden agenda. A thorough explanation of the recovery process and potential risks is necessary and the child should be encouraged to provide written informed consent to further emphasize the gravity of the decision. The parents are still likely to be necessary cosigners even though the patient may be able to consent to some procedures without the parent(s) in some jurisdictions.

As skeletal maturity approaches, some procedures such as epiphysiodesis may be less useful with insufficient growth years remaining to correct deformity. Other proce-dures such as osteotomy and arthrodesis may become safer and even necessary to address joint adaptation. Orthotic and orthodigital treatments are still indicated even after growth plate fusion because path-mechanical abnormalities may continue to deform even mature bones and ligaments. Muscle imbalances always overcome bone structure, even after corrective bone surgery. Bones are plastic and deformable.

SPECIAL NEEDS POPULATIONS

Lower extremity deformities are endemic to many patients with special needs. Over-pronation seems to be the default mechanism of the foot in many patients. A patient with and even mild cognitive disability may, subconsciously, seek better balance with a wider more abducted gate. Congenital deformities may be exacerbated by abnor-malities in muscle tone or ligament molecular integrity. Again, whatever is wrong with the lower extremities is likely to get worse even though the underlying diseases may be chromosomal and/or congenital.

In addition to the tendency for deformity to progress, the child may be unable to voice or describe symptoms. Therefore, it is incumbent on caregivers, coaches, allied treating providers and the specialist to thoroughly examine patients with special needs. A special athlete already has enough obstacles without ill-fitting footwear over painful deformities. Gait examination combined with questioning of people close to the patient may reveal limping. Prompt examination of the patient's feet immediately after exertion may reveal areas of previously unnoticed noxious pressure.

If symptomatic and/or disabling deformity are discovered, management decisions may be difficult. Although the same 4 approaches exist, special concerns regarding appropriate care, consent, and treatment goals also exist. Noninvasive preventative/maintenance approaches seem entirely appropriate even in this austere medical economic environment.

Pain management may be particularly challenging. The patient's ability to report successful treatment and/or negative side effects may be limited. Many of these patients are taking other medications that may interact negatively. Application of invasive pain management treatments such as interarticular injections may be intolerable to a patient with limited ability to understand how to cooperate.

Techniques to induce anesthesia may make surgical treatment relatively easy to complete, but postoperative care may be particularly challenging. The patient's ability to cooperate may be limited. Wounds may be inappropriately handled by the patient. Weight-bearing and operative site elevation restrictions and instructions may not be followed. Wearing prescribed protective postoperative devices may not be complied with well. Precautions such as inpatient care and possibly skilled nursing care may be indicated. Casting may protect surgical incisions, but may increase the risk of deep vein thrombophlebitis, infection, or tight casts. Patients may be unable to describe the symptoms of these potentially serious complications.

Despite this disconcerting list, the risk/benefit ratio may still favor invasive care in some cases. The fact that a patient has special needs should not deny him appropriate treatment. Mitigation of symptoms may be life changing for any patient, opening doors for greater participation in their environment. Employment opportunities, athletic participation (particularly important because many of these populations tend toward obesity), and social and cultural opportunities can be brought into reach.

SUMMARY

Pediatric first ray deformities may present in many ways similar to those affecting adults. However, these patients are not adults. Management of the patient and the deformity necessitates special consideration of timing, the patient's general health, techniques, and perhaps goals. Any simple broad brush approach to the care of these patients will certainly result in both undertreatment and overtreatment. The proper care of these patients is an ongoing process of appropriate management tailored to the patient's needs, deformities, and developmental age. Proper adherence to these recommendations can improve the patient's quality of life and result in a gratifying professional experience for the dedicated health care provider.

REFERENCES

1. Root MI, Orien WP, Weed JH. Normal and abnormal function of the foot. In: Clinical biomechanics, vol. 2. Los Angeles (CA): Clinical Biomechanics; 1977. p. 1–478.

2. Agnew P, Raducanu Y. An algorithmic approach to evaluation of the flatfoot. Clin Podiatr Med Surg 2000;17:383–96.
3. Agnew P. Evaluation of the child with ligamentous laxity. Clin Podiatr Med Surg 1997;14:117–29.
4. Matthew 7:11Good news translation. New York: American Bible Society; 1992.
5. Kalen V, Brecher T. Relationship between adolescent bunions and flat feet. Foot Ankle 1988;8:331–6.
6. Staheli L, Chew DE, Corbett M. The longitudinal arch. J Bone Joint Surg Am 1987; 69:426–8.
7. Kite HJ. The clubfoot. New York: Grune & Stratton; 1964.
8. Tachdjian MO. Pediatric orthopedics, vol. 2. Philadelphia: WB Saunders; 1972. p. 1323.
9. Stark JG, Johanson JE, Winter RB. The Heyman-Herndon tarsometatarsal capsulotomy for metatarsus adductus: results in 48 feet. J Pediatr Orthop 1987;7: 305–10.
10. Lichtblau S. Section of the abductor hallucis tendon for correction of metatarsus adductus varus deformity. Clin Orthop 1975;110:227–32.
11. Joplin R. Sling procedure for correction of splay-foot, metatarsus primus varus, and hallux valgus. J Bone Joint Surg 1950;32:779–92.
12. Holmes G. New procedure straightens bunions without cutting bone. (IL): Rush University Medical Center; 2010. News release.
13. Kayiaros S, Blankenhorn BD, Dehaven J, et al. Correction of metatarsus primus varus associated with hallux valgus deformity using the arthrex mini tightrope: a report of 44 cases. Foot Ankle Spec 2011;4(4):212–7.
14. Driano AN, Staheli L, Staheli LT. Psychosocial development and corrective shoewear use in childhood. J Pediatr Orthop 1998;18(3):346–9.
15. Mahan CC, Mahan KT. Patient preparation in pediatric surgery. Clin Podiatr Med Surg 1987;4(1):1–9.
16. Ellis VH. A method of correcting metatarsus primus varus. J Bone Joint Surg Br 1951;33:415–7.
17. Wenger DR, Mauldin D, Speck G, et al. Corrective shoes and inserts as treatment for flexible flatfoot in infants and children. J Bone Joint Surg Am 1987;71:426–8.

Pediatric Heel Pain

Alison M. Joseph, DPM*, Irene K. Labib, DPM

KEYWORDS

- Heel pain • Pediatric • Trauma • Tumor • Overuse injuries • Calcaneus

KEY POINTS

- Pediatric heel pain may be a common complaint in a podiatrist's office.
- With several possible causes, clinicians must thoroughly evaluate the patient to determine the correct diagnosis.
- Although most causes of heel pain are benign, proper diagnostic tools may be necessary, including radiographs and computed tomography scan.
- The ultimate goal is to allow the child to resume regular activities with no pain.

Heel pain is a common complaint among young children and adolescents. It has several possible causes, including trauma, overuse injuries, and tumors, and therefore a thorough clinical examination is warranted. Gathering a detailed history from the patient and the parent can help clinicians determine the correct diagnosis and treatment plan to allow the child to return to preinjury levels as quickly as possible. This article outlines some common causes of pediatric heel pain.

ANATOMY OF THE CALCANEUS

In any pediatric discussion of heel pain, one must remember the presence of the epiphyseal or growth plate, along with the ossification centers and approximate years of closure. The calcaneus is composed of 2 ossification centers. The primary ossification center is present at birth and located in the calcaneal tuberosity. The secondary ossification center, the apophysis, begins in girls around 4 to 7 years of age and in boys around 7 to 9 years of age. Before the apophysis appears, the posterior calcaneus is irregular, with a saw-tooth appearance (**Fig. 1**).[1] The apophysis develops from multiple centers that coalesce to form one irregular apophysis. Before fusion, the apophysis is more dense than the body of the calcaneus. Fusion of the apophysis to the calcaneus is complete by 15 to 17 years of age.

SEVER DISEASE/CALCANEAL APOPHYSITIS

In 1912, Dr James Warren Sever[2] first described Sever disease or calcaneal apophysitis as a chronic heel pain in the pediatric population. Calcaneal apophysitis is an

Department of Podiatry, University Hospital, 150 Bergen Street, G-142, Newark, NJ 07103, USA
* Corresponding author.
E-mail address: josepham@umdnj.edu

Clin Podiatr Med Surg 30 (2013) 503–511
http://dx.doi.org/10.1016/j.cpm.2013.07.003
0891-8422/13/$ – see front matter © 2013 Elsevier Inc. All rights reserved.

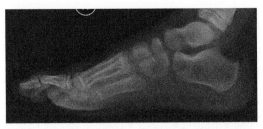

Fig. 1. Saw-tooth appearance of the calcaneus before the appearance of the apophysis.

inflammation of the apophysis caused by the constant pull of the Achilles tendon on the unossified apophysis. Most commonly, children presenting with calcaneal apophysitis are physically active and have an insidious onset of pain. Often the onset coincides with a recent growth spurt, which causes more tension to the area from the stretched Achilles tendon. Calcaneal apophysitis generally presents in boys between 8 and 14 years of age and girls between 8 and 10 years of age.

On clinical evaluation, pain is located directly over the attachment of the Achilles tendon on the calcaneus. Direct side-to-side palpation to the area and surrounding area will elicit pain. Pain can also be noted with active or passive ankle joint dorsiflexion. Rarely, edema or erythema is present in the area. Discomfort is exacerbated by activity and relieved with rest. Many times, the child will refuse to walk on the affected side or walk on the toes to avoid tension on the Achilles tendon. The child may also have difficulty running, jumping, or playing usual sports, and may request frequent breaks or to stop playing. The problem may be bilateral, and until recently was more common in boys.

Calcaneal apophysitis is mainly a clinical diagnosis. Radiographic evaluation is generally unnecessary and occasionally only used to rule out other possible causes. On radiographs the apophysis is irregular with a sclerotic appearance (**Fig. 2**). In 2002, Volpon and Filho[3] investigated the radiographic appearance of the calcaneus in 69 children with calcaneal apophysitis, and 392 children who were asymptomatic. Their data showed that the sclerotic appearance of the apophysis was a normal feature and should not be used to diagnose calcaneal apophysitis. The most

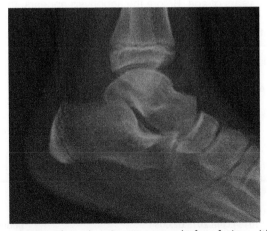

Fig. 2. Irregular apophysis with a sclerotic appearance before fusion with the calcaneus.

significant finding between the groups was that the children with calcaneal apophysitis had a more fragmented apophysis, which they suggested indicated a mechanical cause of the condition (**Fig. 3**).

In 2010, Kose[4] prospectively studied 71 consecutive radiographs of 61 patients diagnosed with calcaneus apophysis. Among these radiographs, 70 were considered to show normal findings. The diagnosis changed in only 1 case, in which a simple bone cyst was present. All patients experienced a positive response to conservative treatment.

Calcaneal apophysitis is self-limiting and will resolve on fusion of the apophysis. Thus, treatment is directed at symptom relief. The child may need to decrease or stop physical or sports activity for a short period until the painful symptoms decrease, which usually occurs after 3 to 4 weeks. Physical therapy may be initiated and is focused on stretching the Achilles tendon. Exercises that stretch the heel cord will help relieve symptoms by taking stress off of the apophysis. Nonsteroidal anti-inflammatory drugs, such as ibuprofen, may also be used to decrease pain and inflammation. In the most severe cases, immobilization in a walking boot or cast for a short period (2–3 weeks) may allow rest and healing. Once the condition has improved, the child should continue a regular stretching regime to prevent recurrence. Surgical intervention is not indicated for calcaneal apophysitis.

BONE TUMORS

Osseous tumors should also be considered in the differential diagnosis. Bone tumors of the calcaneus are rare. The 3 most common bone tumors of the calcaneus are osteoid osteoma, intraosseous lipoma, and unicameral bone cysts. Often patients experience a dull, deep pain in the heel that progresses and is associated with swelling.

Osteoid osteomas are benign bone lesions that are less than 2 cm in diameter. Symptoms include nocturnal pain relieved with salicylates (aspirin). Osteoid osteomas usually present in the first 2 decades of life. Radiographic findings show a round lucent nidus with surrounding dense sclerosis. Osteoid osteoma should be differentiated from Brodie's abscess or localized bone infection. Symptoms will usually last approximately 2.5 years and are often self-limiting. Conservative treatment consists of anti-inflammatory agents and percutaneous computed tomography (CT)–guided radiofrequency coablation.[5–7] Surgical measures include resection of the lesion and bone grafting if pain continues or the size of the lesions causes concern for pathologic fracture.

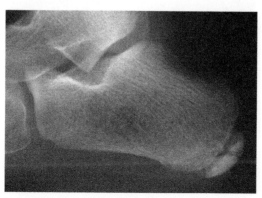

Fig. 3. Fragmented apophysis of a 12-year-old child with calcaneal apophysis.

Unicameral bone cysts are common benign tumors of the calcaneus and usually occur during the first 2 decades of life. They are 2 times more likely to occur in boys than girls.[7] Regarding the rest of the body, the anterior aspect of the calcaneus is the sixth most common location for a unicameral bone cyst to appear (**Fig. 4**).[8] The pathogenesis is indefinite and may be caused by entrapment of synovial tissue[4] or failure of ossification.[9] In most cases, these are diagnosed incidentally based on plain radiographic findings. Unicameral bone cysts appear as radiolucent, circular lesions that do not disrupt the bony cortex.[5] However, in some instances a pathologic fracture can be observed and the "fallen fragment sign" at the base of the lesion is visible on plain films. Because a pathologic fracture is a concern, curettage and bone grafting are part of the treatment protocol.

Intraosseous lipomas constitute approximately 0.1% of all tumors in the body and do not have an age (5–85 years) or sex predilection.[8] The calcaneus is the second most common area where intraosseous lipomas occur, after the femur.[10] Patients will experience intermittent pain in the heel that is aggravated on sporting activities. Symptoms may be caused by the expansion of the lesion, causing remodeling of bone or ischemia within the lesion. On radiographic evaluation, lesions may appear radiolucent or thick and sclerotic, and sometimes resemble a pseudotumor. Other differentials when examining plan films may include osteoblastomas and unicameral bone cysts.[11] Because of the varying appearance of this bone tumor on plain radiographs, advanced imaging is necessary, such as CT or magnetic resonance imaging (MRI). The MRI can differentiate the stages of the bone tumor according to Milgram's Classification.[11] On T1-weighted images the lesion appears sclerotic with surrounding hyperintensity. On T2-weighted images, the fat suppression is visible in the outer periphery, with central area of high signal intensity.[11] Treatments include curettage and bone grafting.

CALCANEAL FRACTURES

Pediatric calcaneal fractures are uncommon injuries, representing less than 0.5% of reported pediatric fractures.[12] Typically, pediatric fractures of the calcaneus are extra-articular and are associated with a low-energy mechanism of injury. Common causes of injury are a fall from a height, motor vehicle accident, or direct blow to the calcaneus.

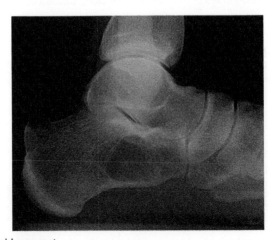

Fig. 4. Unicameral bone cyst.

When a child presents with a suspected calcaneal fracture, standard radiographs are taken of the foot, including anteroposterior, oblique, and lateral views. If a fracture is suspected, a CT is obtained for further evaluation of the fracture. Pediatric calcaneal fractures are classified as either extra-articular or intra-articular. Furthermore, intra-articular fractures can be classified according to the Sanders classification system, which notes the location and degree of comminution through the posterior facet.[13] The Essex-Lopresti classification system may also be used to classify intra-articular calcaneal fractures. On calcaneal impact, a primary fracture line begins at the sinus tarsi and travels either parallel with the plantar foot surface and exits the posterior calcaneus (tongue-type) or separates the posterior facet from the tuberosity as the facet is driven down into the calcaneal body (joint depression).[14]

Historically, all pediatric calcaneal fractures were treated nonoperatively. In current literature the decision to operate is determined by the amount of intra-articular displacement. Many case series have been published reporting good results in children sustaining minimally displaced intra-articular or extra-articular fractures (<2 mm) treated nonoperatively. One report suggested that excellent clinical results are possible with nonoperative treatment, because of many factors, including the potential of the immature talus and calcaneus to grow and remodel post injury, reparative abilities of the surrounding soft tissues, and low-energy trauma causing the fracture.[15]

Mora and colleagues[15] retrospectively reviewed 10 intra-articular and 3 extra-articular fractures of the calcaneus that were treated conservatively. All patients were followed for a minimum of 5 months, with 11 of 12 fractures having good or normal results at final follow-up. One patient with an extra-articular body fracture reported mild ankle pain with physical activity at his final follow-up at 5 months. The investigators further reviewed the long-term results of an additional 8 fractures—6 intra-articular and 2 extra-articular—all treated nonoperatively. At an average of 4.4 years follow-up, 6 of 8 patients scored 68 out of 68 points on the American Orthopaedic Foot and Ankle Score, meaning they had no pain, had unrestricted foot function, had the ability to participate in sports, could walk on uneven surfaces, and had no apparent gait abnormality. Two patients reported mild pain, reducing their score to 58 out of 68. The authors believe the prognosis of pediatric calcaneal fractures is generally satisfactory.[15]

In more recent years, there is a trend toward open reduction and internal fixation for intra-articular fractures with greater than 2 mm of displacement. In 2007, Petit and colleagues[16] retrospectively reviewed 14 fractures in 13 children with intra-articular fractures of the calcaneus with greater than 2 mm displacement. They found that all patients had a good clinical outcome with few complications. Pickle and colleagues[17] in 2004 retrospectively reviewed 7 fractures in 6 children with displaced intra-articular calcaneal fractures, noting no intraoperative or postoperative complications. At a mean follow-up of 9.7 months, all children were pain-free when performing activities of daily living, were able to return to full activity, and had normal ankle range of motion.

Although pediatric calcaneal fractures remain rare, if suspected they must be evaluated and treated appropriately. The goals of treatment are the same as for adult calcaneal fractures: restore the articular surfaces, maintain calcaneal width and height, and restore the lateral wall of the calcaneus.

PEDIATRIC CALCANEAL OSTEOMYELITIS

Although uncommon in children, calcaneus bone infection must be included in the differential diagnosis of pediatric heel pain. The incidence of acute calcaneal osteomyelitis in the pediatric population has been reported to be 3% to 10%.[18] Calcaneal osteomyelitis in children can result from either direct inoculation or acute hematogenous spread. It has a less-dramatic presentation than long bone osteomyelitis, and thus diagnosis is often delayed. Complications include chronic infection, growth arrest, and limb length discrepancy.[19]

Direct inoculation of bacteria causing calcaneal osteomyelitis may occur from a puncture wound, an overlying ulceration, a laceration, or an open injury. Puncture wounds are commonly seen in the emergency department and have a 1.8% incidence of causing calcaneal osteomyelitis in the pediatric population (**Fig. 5**).[20] Infecting organisms include both gram-positive and gram-negative bacteria, but *Pseudomonas aeruginosa* is most commonly associated with puncture wound osteomyelitis.[20]

Acute hematogenous osteomyelitis (AHO) in children most commonly follows bacteremia from another source. Although the infection usually seeds from the respiratory tract, it can also come from the aural, cutaneous, gastrointestinal, and gastrointestinal tracts.[21] Therefore, the family must be questioned regarding recent illness or infections so that a possible cause of pain is not missed.

Signs and symptoms of AHO of the calcaneus may be less dramatic than those for long bones, making diagnosis difficult. Clinical symptoms include pain, toe walking, inability to bear weight, and limping on the affected side. Wang and colleagues[22] described the "heel up" sign, which they believed was diagnostic for calcaneus osteomyelitis. They believe children with infection versus other calcaneus abnormalities will not allow the limb to come in contact with the bed, even during sleep. Clinical signs may also be nonspecific, and include edema, erythema, calor, and point tenderness.

If AHO is suspected, standard procedure includes ordering a white blood cell (WBC) count with differential and blood cultures, and taking the child's temperature. The literature has reported that up to 50% of children may be afebrile, have a mild or no elevation of WBC count, and have negative blood culture results, making early diagnosis difficult.[21] Erythrocyte sedimentation rate (ESR) and C-reactive protein (CRP) are nonspecific markers of inflammation and infection, respectively, that may

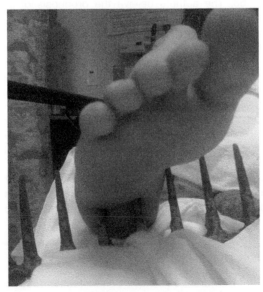

Fig. 5. Direct inoculation osteomyelitis from a puncture wound.

be elevated in AHO. Jaakola and Kehl[18] reported an average delay of 13.1 days in diagnosing calcaneal osteomyelitis in 21 cases. Similarly, Leigh an colleagues[19] noted that 38 of 60 patients were diagnosed on admission to the hospital with AHO, whereas the remaining patients had a delay of 2.9 days because more-sophisticated diagnostic studies were required.

Radiographs of the foot should also be obtained at presentation. Importantly, radiographic changes associated with osteomyelitis are not seen for 7 to 14 days after the onset of infection. Therefore, a bone scan, CT scan, or MRI may be obtained for diagnosis. The gold standard in diagnosing calcaneal osteomyelitis is a bone biopsy.

Treatment of acute hematogenous includes intravenous antibiotic therapy until the inflammatory markers (ESR, CRP) and acute symptoms have resolved, usually within 1 to 2 weeks. Patients should then be switched to oral antibiotics for an additional 2 to 4 weeks. In total, 4 to 6 weeks of antibiotics are recommended in the literature. If the child is not experiencing a response to antibiotics, surgical intervention may be warranted, including incision and drainage, curettage of bone, and possible implantation of antibiotic beads.

RETAINED FOREIGN BODY

The presence of foreign material is often difficult to diagnose in the young pediatric population. Approximately 38% of foreign bodies are missed on initial presentation.[23] A detailed history from the parent/guardian is imperative. Inquiry as to whether shoe gear was involved is necessary to determine the level of contamination and the presence of shoe materials, such as leather or rubber. Puncture wounds and retained foreign bodies mostly occur in warm environments because of increased outdoor activity and ambulation without shoe gear.

The child may complain of point tenderness at a specific area on the plantar aspect of the heel and be unable to weight-bear. Depending on the acuteness of the injury, evidence of the puncture may be visible or overlying hyperkeratosis can be seen. The most common culprits of puncture wounds are glass, wood splinters, and metal,[24] such as needles, staples, or shredded metal. Other less-common materials are pencil lead and fishhooks. Pencil lead may cause tattoo-colored pigmentation. Fishhooks can be problematic because of the barbs at the tip; techniques such as insertion of an 18-gauge needle over the barb can facilitate removal.

In the acute emergency room setting, appropriate tetanus prophylaxis is warranted. If concomitant cellulitis is present, the appropriate antibiotic should be initiated. Radiographic imaging can help diagnose the cause if the foreign material is metal because of its radio-opacity. Wood splinters and glass are radiolucent and will not be visible on radiographic films. Other imaging techniques are ultrasonography or CT scan. A metallic marker can be used to assist in localizing the foreign body. If the puncture by the foreign body is longstanding, osseous involvement should be considered and osteomyelitis must be ruled out. If removal of the foreign material is attempted, sedation along with local anesthesia may be necessary. Discontinuing the attempt to remove the foreign material after 30 minutes[25] is important to avoid damage to underlying structures or burying the material deeper within the soft tissue. Operative management at that point may be necessary to evacuate the foreign body and drain an abscess that may have formed to wall off the foreign material. In a study by Huurman and Bhuller,[26] cast immobilization allowed for foreign body extrusion after failed initial exploration. This technique represents an alternative to surgical removal and exploration of retained radiolucent foreign material if no underlying infection is present.

SUMMARY

Pediatric heel pain may be a common complaint in a podiatrist's office. With several possible causes, a thorough evaluation is important to determine the correct diagnosis. Although most of the causes of heel pain are benign, proper diagnostic tools may be necessary, including radiographs and CT scan. The ultimate goal is to allow the child to resume regular activities with no pain.

REFERENCES

1. Logan AL. The foot and ankle: clinical applications. Gaithersburg (MD): Aspen Publisher; 1995.
2. Sever JW. Apophysitis of the os calsis. NY Med J 1912;95:1025–9.
3. Volpon JB, Filho G. Calcaneal apophysitis: a quantitative radiographic evaluation of the secondary ossification center. Arch Orthop Trauma Surg 2002;122:338–41.
4. Kose O. Do we really need radiologic assessment for the diagnosis of non-specific heel pain (calcaneal apophysitis) in children. Skeletal Radiol 2010; 39:359–61.
5. Jay R. 1st edition. Pediatric foot and ankle surgery, vol. 2. Philadelphia: Saunders Co; 1999.
6. Saraph V, Zwick E, Maizen C, et al. Treatment of unicameral calcaneal bone cysts in children: review of literature and results using a cannulated screw for continuous decompression of the cyst. J Pediatr Ophthalmol 2004;24:568–73.
7. Mirra JL. 1st edition. Bone tumors, vol. 20. Philadelphia: Lea & Febiger; 1989.
8. Propeck T, Bullard MA, Lin J, et al. Radiologic-pathologic correlation of intraosseous lipomas. AJR Am J Roentgenol 2000;175:673–8.
9. Jaffe JL, Lichtenstein L. Solitary unicameral bone cyst with emphasis on the roentgen picture, the pathologic appearance and the pathogenesis. Arch Surg 1942;44:1004–25.
10. Murphey M, Carroll J, Flemming D, et al. From the archives of the AFIP: benign musculoskeletal lipomatous lesions. Radiographics 2004;24:1433–66.
11. Milgram JW. Intraosseous lipomas: radiologic and pathologic manifestations. Radiology 1988;167:155–60.
12. Wiley JJ, Profitt A. Fractures of the os calsis in children. Clin Orthop 1984;188: 131–8.
13. Sanders R. Intra-articular fractures of the calcaneus: present state of the art. J Orthop Trauma 1992;6(2):254.
14. Essex-Lopresti P. The mechanism, reduction technique, and results in fractures of the os calsis. Br J Surg 1952;39:395–419.
15. Mora S, Thordarson DB, Zionts LE, et al. Pediatric calcaneal fractures. Foot Ankle Int 2001;22:471–7.
16. Petit CJ, Lee BM, Kasser JR, et al. Operative treatment of intraarticular calcaneal fractures in the pediatric population. J Pediatr Orthop 2007;27:856–62.
17. Pickle AP, Benaroch TE, Guy P, et al. Clinical outcome of pediatric calcaneal fractures treated with open reduction and internal fixation. J Pediatr Orthop 2004;24:178–80.
18. Jaakola JL, Kehl D. Hematogenous calcaneal osteomyelitis in children. J Pediatr Orthop 1999;19:699–704.
19. Leigh W, Crawford H, Street M, et al. Pediatric calcaneal osteomyelitis. J Pediatr Orthop 2010;30:888–92.
20. Cetinus E, Ciragil P, Penninick A. Calcaneal osteomyelitis after puncture wound to foot: case report and review of the literature. J Orthop Trauma 2005;6:194–6.

21. O'Shea MK, Still G, Bledsoe CA. Laboratory considerations in the surgical treatment of acute hematogenous osteomyelitis of the calcaneus. J Foot Ankle Surg 1998;37:148–55.

22. Wang EH, Simpson S, Bennet G. Osteomyelitis of the calcaneum. J Bone Joint Surg Br 1992;74:906–9.

23. Anderson MA, Newmeyer WL 3rd, Kilgore ES Jr. Diagnosis and treatment of retained foreign bodies in the hand. Am J Surg 1982;144(1):63–7.

24. Levine MR, Gorman SM, Young CF, et al. Clinical characteristics and management of wound foreign bodies in the ED. Am J Emerg Med 2008;26(8): 918–22.

25. Chiodo WA, Cook KD. Pediatric heel pain. Clin Podiatr Med Surg 2010;27(3): 355–67.

26. Huurman W, Bhuller G. Nonoperative treatment of retained radiolucent foreign bodies in lower limbs. J Pediatr Orthop 1982;2(5):506–8.

Treatment of the Neglected and Relapsed Clubfoot

Harold Jacob Pieter van Bosse, MD[a,b,]*

KEYWORDS

- Clubfoot • Relapse • Neglected • Ilizarov • Ponseti • Foot osteotomies

KEY POINTS

- Tibialis anterior tendon transfers help rebalance relapsed clubfeet but only feet that are passively correctable.
- Extensive soft tissue releases for clubfoot relapse have a high rate of recurrence; the results are better in older children than in younger ones.
- The Evans and Lichtblau procedures lead to subtalar stiffness and gradual deterioration of results over time.
- Osteotomies across the cuneiform-cuboid axis only correct forefoot deformities and do not address hindfoot varus.
- Neglected and severe relapsed clubfeet can be corrected gradually with external fixators.
  - Correcting with osteotomies and external fixators has a high rate of recurrence.
  - Using external fixators for gradual correction after soft tissue releases does not provide consistent results.
  - Soft tissue distraction with an external fixator allows for clubfoot correction with decreased risks of neurovascular injury and a lower rate of recurrence.
- The Ponseti method of serial casting is a valid treatment option for nearly all neglected and relapsed clubfeet, except for those with bony synostoses or arthrodeses.

DEFINITION OF NEGLECTED AND RELAPSED CLUBFOOT

Idiopathic clubfoot deformities are the most common musculoskeletal congenital abnormalities. Treatment in much of the world has become standardized around the Ponseti technique. There are still several problems to be solved within the topic of clubfoot treatment—among the most challenging is the neglected and relapsed clubfoot.

Disclosures: No funding sources or conflicts of interest.
[a] Shriners Hospital for Children, Department of Orthopaedic Surgery, 3551 North Broad Street, Philadelphia, PA 19140, USA; [b] Department of Orthopaedic Surgery, Temple University, Philadelphia, PA
* Corresponding author. Shriners Hospital for Children, Department of Orthopaedic Surgery, 3551 North Broad Street, Philadelphia, PA 19140, USA.
E-mail address: HvanBosse@Shrinenet.org

Clin Podiatr Med Surg 30 (2013) 513–530
http://dx.doi.org/10.1016/j.cpm.2013.07.006
0891-8422/13/$ – see front matter © 2013 Elsevier Inc. All rights reserved.

podiatric.theclinics.com

Ponseti stated, "regardless of the mode of treatment, the clubfoot has a stubborn tendency to relapse."[1] The rate of relapse is estimated between 10% and 50% regardless of the mode of initial correction used.[2–5] Proposed causes of deformity recurrence break into 2 groups: undercorrection[2,6] and continued activation of the primary factors that created the clubfoot initially.[1] The primary factors include muscle imbalances[7] and myofibroblasts in the medial fascia,[8,9] although presence of the latter has been disputed.[10] Contributing factors include postsurgical scarring and the underutilization of post-treatment bracing.[3,11] This review only considers relapses with elements of a clubfoot: equinus, heel varus, midfoot supination, cavus, and forefoot adductus. Relapsed feet with other deformities, such as severe heel valgus and/or forefoot abductus (the overcorrected clubfoot), or with a midfoot break (rockerbottom) are not discussed.

The definition of a neglected clubfoot is somewhat ill defined. There is a commonly understood social implication of neglect, similar to child neglect, where timely attention is not paid to the foot deformity. This definition varies with local cultural norms and expectancies of when a child's parents should seek treatment to avoid developmental delays, ambulation difficulties, and shoe wear problems. This article is more interested in a medical definition, in which a neglected clubfoot is not treated until after the age when the usual treatments are expected to produce a successful deformity correction. Turco[12,13] stated that his release was optimally performed between 1 and 2 years of age, but the upper limit was 6 years of age. Simons[14,15] noted that he had no minimum age but thought that the foot should be a minimum of 8 cm in length; he thought that his release was best suited for children less than 4 years of age. Although Ponseti did not express an upper age limit for successful application of his technique, he only reported on babies whose treatment was initiated before 6 months of age.[1,4,5,16] Subsequent reports have documented that the Ponseti method can be used to correct an initially untreated clubfoot well past the age of 12 months.[17–22] So, within an expanded age range, an obviously neglected clubfoot to one practitioner may be seen as merely a more challenging foot to another.

What makes a neglected or relapsed clubfoot different and more difficult to treat compared with a newborn's clubfoot? First, the feet are stiffer. The capsular tissues have hypertrophied with growth and weight bearing. In cases of previous surgical release, there is an element of thick scar formation. Second, the tarsal bones are further matured. The tarsal bones in an infant are largely, if not wholly, composed of cartilage, and correction of a clubfoot at this age occurs in part through morphologic changes of the cartilaginous bones as they respond to newer, more physiologic stresses.[1,23] Third, weight bearing may create trophic changes, such as skin callosities and mild bony hypertrophy at the site of impact, with hypoplasia of the correspondingly understressed structures. Fourth, there is theoretically an acclimation of the abnormally positioned muscles and tendons to the long-standing deformity. In the neglected clubfoot, for example, the abductor hallucis muscle becomes a powerful force maintaining forefoot supination and cavus; the tibialis anterior muscle becomes strong with hypertrophied tendon, whereas its antagonists, the peronei muscles, are overstretched and weak.

The goal of treating a neglected or relapsed clubfoot is the same as for a newborn's clubfoot: a plantigrade, flexible foot, which is pain-free, normal looking, and requiring no shoe modifications,[1,24] with the least chance for relapse. Although plantigrade is nearly always an achievable goal, flexible is more difficult because the foot usually is stiff at the onset. Interventions should be chosen with an eye toward preventing further intracapsular scarring or bony fusions, when possible. In addition, several treatment options shorten an already small foot, so there should be emphasis on maintaining the length of the foot as best possible. The goals of patients need to be considered as well. Salinas and colleagues[25] describe a 30-year-old woman with an untreated clubfoot, bearing weight over the dorsum of the foot and wearing a high-topped shoe backwards. She did not complain of pain or functional impairment and only inadvertently came to medical attention when seeking treatment for her 18-month-old son with his congenital clubfoot.

SOFT TISSUE PROCEDURES

Soft tissue procedures can be appropriate treatment of the relapsed clubfoot, especially with mild deformities, but are unlikely to adequately correct a neglected clubfoot. A common cause of clubfoot relapses is muscular imbalance across the forefoot.[7,26] In many instances, the ability of the peroneal muscles to pronate/evert is fundamentally impaired and is overpowered by the otherwise normally functioning tibialis anterior muscle. During the swing-through portion of gait, the unopposed pull of the tibialis anterior leads to supination/inversion rather than dorsiflexion, causing the foot to be prepositioned for foot strike along the lateral forefoot. An effective correction for this dynamic problem is the transfer of the tibialis anterior tendon. Garceau[26] initially described the procedure for recurrent clubfeet in 1940, anchoring the transferred tendon to the proximal end of the fifth metatarsal. In a review of 22 feet of 19 patients at an average of 15 years after transfer, Garceau and Palmer[27] found that the majority had a good to excellent gait patterns, although some of the feet "had a very mild planovalgus deformity" and 1 patient had "extreme planovalgus deformity" bilaterally. Ponseti found that most repeatedly relapsing clubfeet responded well to transfer of the tibialis anterior tendon, often along with a tendoachilles tenotomy, but only after 2.5 years of age.[5] Of the 94 feet in Ponseti and Smoley's[5] first description of the serial casting method, 38 required transfer of the tibialis anterior; of those, only 1 required a subsequent medial release. Initially, the tendon was transferred to either the third cuneiform or the cuboid, but later reports only described a transfer to the third cuneiform; no cases of overcorrection into planovalgus were reported on follow-up.[1,5,28] Prior to transferring the tendon, the foot needed to be supple enough that it could be passively corrected; if it was not, it should first undergo serial casting to achieve the corrected position prior to tendon transfer. Kuo and colleagues[29] reported on 71 tibialis anterior tendon transfers for clubfoot relapse (presumably after surgical correction). Full tendon transfers to the middle or the third cuneiform were done in 42 feet, whereas 27 feet underwent a split tendon transfer, with the transferred lateral half anchored to the cuboid. They found that the full transfer had a slightly better correction of the forefoot supination, as measured radiographically, but that the split transfer had better retained inversion strength; these differences were clinically insignificant. Farsetti and colleagues[30] found that the clinical results were better for tendon transfers performed on post–Ponseti casting relapsed clubfeet compared with those feet that had their initial correction by posterior-medial releases. Of those with postsurgical relapses, feet that were passively correctable had a better result compared with feet too stiff to passively correct. None of the patients had further relapses. Plain radiographs and CT scans showed that the cuneiforms and cuboid were laterally shifted due to the tendon transfer, which did not seem to compromise the functional results. Transfer of the tibialis posterior through the intraosseous membrane to the dorsum of the foot has also been proposed, but indications for this procedure for clubfoot relapse are probably limited to instances of drop foot, because this procedure is more invasive and the transfer is out of phase.[1,31]

For stiffer and more severe relapses, soft tissue releases have been proposed. Park and colleagues[32] reported on a series of 19 clubfeet that relapsed after Ponseti casting and were treated with an à la carte strategy of selective surgeries. Procedures included combinations of Achilles, tibialis posterior and/or tibialis anterior lengthening, abductor hallucis muscle release, plantar fasciotomy, and medial joint capsulotomy. Despite the surgeries, approximately 50% required another surgery at a mean follow-up of 2.7 years. Bensahel and colleagues[33] used their physical therapy method for clubfoot correction and described a different à la carte approach for 142 relapsed feet. Through a medial incision, the abductor hallucis muscle was released, the tibialis posterior tendon Z-lengthened, and the talonavicular joint released, with pinning of the joint. Then posteriorly, the tibiotalar joint capsule was incised, the Achilles lengthened, and the lateral subtalar joint was apparently released. At a mean 8.5-years' follow-up, they reported 88% good results. Bost and colleagues[34] used a medially based incision to perform an extensive plantar dissection, with complete release of the abductor halluces muscle, plantar intrinsic muscles, and the tibialis posterior tendon, along with a plantar fasciotomy. Also, complete capsulotomies effected a circumferential release of the navicular, the subtalar joint, and the plantar calcaneocuboid joint. Once the surgical incisions healed, the patients would often undergo progressive deformity correction through serial casting for an average of 5.5 months; 70 feet underwent the procedure at an average age of 6.7 years, and, at an average of 7.5 years' follow-up, approximately half had good to excellent results, but approximately half had required subsequent procedures. Sherman and Westin[35] had a similar but much less invasive treatment, with a plantar release through a short lateral incision, followed by serial casting every 2 weeks—101 feet were treated by this method at a mean age of 8.9 years, one-third were neglected clubfeet, and the others were postsurgical relapses; 97% of children 6 years of age or older had a satisfactory result and required no further procedures, but only 53% for children less than 6 years of age were satisfactory.

Several investigators have advocated the conventional complete clubfoot soft tissue release for acute correction of the neglected or relapsed foot, addressing the main concern of the skin closure viability in differing ways. Various incisions have been suggested to alleviate tension across the closure, such as a double (medial and a posterolateral) zigzag incision,[36] a nearly circumferential incision over the dorsum of the foot,[37] an anteromedial foot and ankle–based fasciocutaneous rotational flap,[38] and an extensive incision from the neck of the first metatarsal to the midcalf.[39] The numbers of patients presented in these studies were small, but the incisions reportedly all healed primarily. Other than a series of children with Moebius syndrome with a 67% recurrence rate,[39] outcomes of these studies were poorly defined, stating only that further surgeries were rarely needed. Hassan and colleagues[40] favored a cross-leg flap to cover the medial and posterior skin deficits after a complete subtalar release, with transection of the flap pedicle at 3 weeks; 30 feet were treated at a mean age of 5.6 years and only 1 incision developed marginal necrosis, which healed by secondary intention after débridement. The radiographic and patient satisfaction outcomes at a mean of 4.5 years were reportedly good. A few small studies examined the use of tissue expanders to aid in skin closure for a subsequent clubfoot soft tissue release, with mixed results.[41,42] The procedures were done for young children, approximately half under 12 months of age. Complication rates were 20% to 70%, primarily infections and skin necrosis; outcomes of the clubfoot procedures were not given.

BONE PROCEDURES

One of the main differences between soft tissue procedures and most bone procedures is that the latter shorten the foot, whereas the soft tissue releases by and large do not. As such, bone procedures are often used for more severe deformities, especially those that are stiffer or have skin coverage issues. Tarraf and Carroll[6] documented that with every subsequent procedure to treat a recurrent relapse, the foot was more likely to undergo a bony procedure. In their study, first reoperations were treated solely with soft tissue procedures in 26% of cases, whereas none of the feet requiring a second or third reoperation was treated only by soft tissue releases. Although a triple arthrodesis is one of the oldest bone procedures for clubfoot correction, it is certainly a procedure of last resort.[43,44] The challenge is to balance deformity correction with maintenance of flexibility and foot length.

Evans[45] described a procedure that combined a posteromedial release with a lateral column shortening by way of resecting and fusing the calcaneocuboid joint. He reasoned that with further growth, the tethered lateral column would resist recurrence into adductus. To avoid growth-related overcorrection, he recommended delaying surgery until after 6 years of age by casting and bracing, even in virgin clubfeet.[46] Fortunately, there are 2 long-term follow-up studies on Evans' own patients. Tayton and Thompson[47] found that at an average follow-up of 10.7 years, 78% of the 84 patients had good and fair functional results but that hindfoot motion was severely limited in 50% and slightly limited in another 43%. Graham and Dent[48] were able to evaluate 45 patients from that last study at an average follow-up of 23 years, noting that the functional good and fair results had decreased to 68%, with 23% of the feet having developed adductus and 12% having undergone triple arthrodeses. Severe hindfoot valgus and planus feet were described in a few cases. In order to maintain hindfoot motion and prevent the growth-related problems of the Evans procedure, Lichtblau[49] modified the procedure, also performing an extensive release but only resecting the anterior process of the calcaneus, creating a pseudojoint with the unaltered cuboid. At an average of 3 years' follow-up, of the 13 feet, Lichtblau[49] found 6 had fair or poor results, which he considered "encouraging." Mehrafshan and colleagues[50] reported on a series of children undergoing procedures for relapsed clubfeet, in which 65% of feet undergoing the Lichtblau procedure had severe subtalar stiffness, and 23% had moderate stiffness.

Many procedures have been described for clubfoot relapses as variations on a theme, obtaining correction across the cuneiform-cuboid axis of the foot. These include a medial cuneiform opening wedge osteotomy (with a radical plantar release and tibialis anterior transfer) to correct cavus and adductus[51]; a medial cuneiform opening wedge and cuboid closing wedge osteotomy for more aggressive adductus correction[52,53]; a medial cuneiform opening wedge and cuboid closing wedge osteotomy, completing the midfoot osteotomy through the other 2 cuneiforms, to allow for more supination correction[54]; a medial cuneiform opening wedge and cuboid closing wedge osteotomy with a dorsally based wedge resection of the other 2 cuneiforms, for more aggressive cavus correction[55]; and a transverse osteotomy through the cuneiforms (without an opening wedge) and a closing wedge cuboid osteotomy.[56] All the procedures were done for the so-called bean-shaped foot, with adductus and supination of the forefoot. All the investigators claimed high rates of success, in terms of patient and parent satisfaction with the foot shape. All documented correction of the talo–first metatarsal angle anywhere from 9° to 28° — the more tarsal bones osteotomized, the greater the correction. Some of the patients were as young as 2.5 years old at the time of the procedure, but most were over 4 years old, recommended as a minimum age for the osteotomies so that the ossific nucleus of the medial cuneiform is well formed.[53] I find that the osteotomies along the cuneiform-cuboid axis are beneficial for more minor residual deformities, but there are several caveats. First, as Davidson[57] pointed out, midfoot procedures that did not osteotomize the middle and lateral cuneiform have to pivot through the second and third tarsal-metatarsal joints, which have to be wedged into valgus. Second, the corrections obtained are off-axis, because the actual deformity is at the Chopart joint. Farsetti and colleagues[58] demonstrated that the navicular was medially subluxated on the talus in 75% to 90% of CT scans of adults' feet after successful clubfoot treatment as infants. Therefore, the osteotomies create a second deformity to compensate for a malalignment that is still present. Third, as is the flaw with many studies of pediatric conditions, the follow-up is short, averaging 2 to 4.5 years, and few patients were followed to skeletal maturity. One of the patients with the longest follow-up was essentially pain-free for 10 years, but at 21 years of age she required a triple arthrodesis.[54] Fourth, the osteotomies only correct the forefoot/midfoot findings of adductus and possibly supination and cavus but do not address hindfoot varus. Some of the studies admitted as much,[52,55] whereas others either stated that none of their patients had heel varus[53] or that the varus was corrected by their particular type of midfoot osteotomy.[56] Hofmann and colleagues[51] addressed the heel varus by performing a medial release along with the medial cuneiform opening wedge osteotomy, but they did not report whether the heel positioning was subsequently corrected.

Dwyer[59,60] described a medial calcaneal opening wedge osteotomy to correct residual hindfoot varus. By remaining extra-articular, he reasoned that flexibility could be preserved. Occasionally, he combined this osteotomy with one at the tarsometatarsal level to correct forefoot supination or adductus. In a review of 36 feet on which Dwyer had operated, at a 27-year mean follow-up, Kumar and colleagues[61] found excellent results in 94%, although 2 heels were still in varus, and 14 were apparently in excessive but nonsymptomatic valgus. Lundberg[62] reported his results on 29 feet, with more than half the patients younger than 2 years old; the youngest was 3 months. Approximately 80% of the cases were satisfactory, but the unsatisfactory cases were equally divided between lack of correction and valgus overcorrection.[62] One caveat of that study was a 40% rate of partial wound edge necrosis.

Several other bony procedures have been proposed. Souchet and colleagues[63] obtained rotational correction of the calcaneoforefoot unit without violating the subtalar joint, to normalize a low anteroposterior talocalcaneal angle on radiograph. They performed a combined medial and plantar soft tissue release, in part to mobilize the talonavicular joint, then created a crescentic calcaneal osteotomy just below the subtalar joint, allowing the foot to rotate under the talus through the osteotomy; 21 procedures were done at an average age of 7 years, and at 2.8 years' follow-up, the talocalcaneal angle had normalized. The talonavicular joint was well reduced in 18 feet but dorsally displaced in 2. There was no mention of whether the heel varus was corrected. Napiontek and Nazar[64] used a compensatory tibial osteotomy to create a plantigrade foot. Derotational osteotomies were used to correct medial malalignment syndrome (inturning of the foot in comparison with the knee), or biplanar or triplanar supramalleolar osteotomies were used to compensate residual equinus, varus and/or internal rotation of the foot. At a mean of 4.3 years, 8 of 19 feet did not have an improvement in their deformity. The investigators stated that there are exceptionally rare indications for the procedure. They also agreed with those who did not believe internal tibial torsion is associated with the clubfoot deformity, a finding further proved by CT scan studies.[65]

Although most of these series related primarily to relapsed clubfeet, a few studies addressed bony procedures for neglected clubfeet. el-Tayeby[66] reported on 28 neglected clubfeet in patients between 4 and 14 years of age.[66] After an extensive posteromedial soft tissue release, he would perform a trapezoidal cuboid resectional osteotomy, transfer the tibialis anterior to the cuboid, and, in 28%, a Dwyer osteotomy of the calcaneus. After a 26-month average follow-up, 89% of the feet had satisfactory results, because by the Abrams classification,[67] the 39% fair results were also considered satisfactory. He found that neither patient age nor severity of deformity was significantly associated with unsatisfactory results. Herold and Torok[68] described a 2-staged operation on 44 feet of older children and adults. The first stage was an extensive medial release, including sectioning of the tibialis posterior, followed by serial casting to obtain maximal correction. The second stage was a triple arthrodesis, and in 50% supplemental procedures were done for residual deformities. At 2- to 6-year follow-up, 43 feet had good or satisfactory appearance and 38 had good or satisfactory function. Lui[69] presented a case report of a 40-year-old man with a neglected clubfoot, who underwent an arthroscopic triple arthrodesis, with good cosmetic results; no functional results were reported. Sobel and colleagues[70] performed an extensive plantarfascial and medial release, along with a talonavicular and calcaneocuboid joint resection and arthrodesis on 3 adult patients over 30 years of age with neglected clubfeet (2 of the feet had undergone casting as infants but recurred early in childhood). All patients were pleased with their foot shape, although 2 of the 3 had equinus, and 1 had pain with prolonged ambulation.

Talectomies are often discussed as salvage for severe clubfoot relapses or neglected cases, although the procedure is more commonly used for posttraumatic deformities and after failed procedures for ankle arthritis.[71] Cooper and Capello[72] followed up 26 feet an average of 20 years after having undergone a talectomy at an average age of 10.5 years. Only 4 procedures were done for congenital clubfeet, and the results were not parsed by diagnosis. The talectomy produced a painless, stable foot, with 92% satisfactory results. The investigators recommended that this "drastic procedure" be used only for rigid and severe foot deformities in patients too young for a triple arthrodesis. Legaspi and colleagues[73] reviewed 24 feet that had undergone talectomies for recurrent equinovarus deformities, of which only 1 was idiopathic; the remainder were arthrogryposis or myelomeningocele. At a mean 20-year follow-up, the grouped results were good in 33%, fair in 42% (required further procedures but had a painless gait), and poor in 25%. Mirzayan and colleagues[74] reported on 7 adult feet that had undergone talectomies, 4 of which had neglected clubfeet. The procedure also included tibiocalcaneal, calcaneocuboid, and tibionavicular arthrodeses. Follow-up was only 9 months, but all patients were satisfied with the procedure and would have chosen it again, despite a stiff foot and 3.5-cm average limb shortening.

CORRECTION FACILITATED BY EXTERNAL FIXATORS

Grill and Franke[75] and Franke and colleagues[76] accredited the Russian authors, Abal'masova and Konjuchov, as first describing the use of the Ilizarov external fixator to correcting severe clubfoot relapses in the 1970s. Since then, external fixators have been used to correct these deformities, either in conjunction with soft tissues releases or osteotomies or through soft tissue distraction. Universally, the articles described use of circular fixators, usually Ilizarov frames or Taylor Spatial Frames.

There are 5 principal osteotomies used in concert with external fixators for correcting neglected or residual clubfoot deformities. The first 2 are named for the shape of the bone cuts when viewing the foot laterally.[77–80] The U osteotomy is a crescentic bone cut largely in the body of the calcaneus just below the subtalar joint, cutting across the neck of the talus anteriorly, and exits posteriorly at the superior aspect of the calcaneal tuberosity, just inferior/posterior to the posterior facet. It is useful for cases of talar deformity or when the hindfoot and forefoot align well with each other (eg, hindfoot varus with forefoot supination) and can be repositioned as a unit. The V osteotomy is a double osteotomy, with both limbs starting dorsally similar to the U osteotomy (talar neck anteriorly and just posterior to the subtalar joint posteriorly), converging to an apex on the plantar aspect of the neck of the calcaneus. The V osteotomy allows for correction of the hindfoot and the forefoot separately. The third, the midfoot osteotomy, preserves subtalar motion and is variably described as across the cuneiform-cuboid axis or through the neck of the talus similar to the anterior limb of the V osteotomy. The fourth, the posterior calcaneal osteotomy, is essentially a reverse Koutsogiannis osteotomy[81] across the calcaneal tuberosity, for correcting hindfoot deformities. Lastly, a supramalleolar osteotomy has been used for cases of ankle arthrodesis, with or without talar or subtalar deformities. Paley[79] reported his results treating 25 severe foot deformities with osteotomies and gradual correction with an Ilizarov frame, of which 5 were severe clubfoot relapses. Ages were not given. Deformity correction was complicated in 4 of the 5 clubfeet by 3 premature consolidations (U osteotomy, posterior calcaneal osteotomy, and midfoot osteotomy) and 1 incomplete subtalar osteotomy, all requiring reosteotomies. Despite the midfoot osteotomy healing in supination, the results of all 5 feet were rated satisfactory. Lamm and colleagues[82] stated that osteotomies were essential for any child 8 years of age or older, whereas El-Mowafi and colleagues[83] reserved osteotomies for children older than 10 years of age and only if there was abnormal bony morphology. In the latter study, 16 clubfeet underwent V osteotomies, with an age range of 11 to 29 years. At an average 5.6 years' follow-up, 7 of the 16 feet had recurrent or residual deformity, 3 of which required revision osteotomies and 1 a triple arthrodesis. None, however, had pain at final follow-up.[83] Kocaoğlu and colleagues[78] treated 2 clubfeet with osteotomies and an Ilizarov frame; a 6-year-old patient with a neglected clubfoot had a recurrence but a 13-year-old patient with a relapsed clubfoot remained plantigrade at 24 months' follow-up. Segev and colleagues[84] reported on 8 idiopathic clubfeet that underwent V osteotomy at an average age of 11 years, with a 3.8-year average follow-up. The investigators noted that foot shape and patient satisfaction were significantly improved, but there was no improvement in pain, range of motion, or function. Utukuri and colleagues[85] treated 9 clubfeet at an average 9 years of age with 3 V osteotomies, 2 calcaneal osteotomies, and 4 midfoot osteotomies. At approximately 4 years' average follow-up, only 4 of the 9 feet were plantigrade, and only 3 rated their satisfaction as good or excellent. Finally, Eidelman and colleagues[86] reported on 12 residual clubfoot deformities in children, average age 14.4 years, treated with a midfoot osteotomy using a percutaneous Gigli saw, and obtaining gradual correction with the Taylor Spatial Frame in the Butt frame configuration. Three patients had residual hindfoot varus, of whom 2 underwent calcaneal osteotomies at the time of frame removal. At an average follow-up of just over 3 years, all but 2 patients had good or excellent functional results, although 2 feet required repeat operations. Altogether, this collection of patients who underwent osteotomies to facilitate their clubfoot deformity correction with an Ilizarov external fixator is small, and the results are mixed. They belong within a larger group of complex foot deformities that have been treated in this manner, whose investigators have overall been pleased with the success of the technique.[77,79,82,87] Given the high rates of recurrence or residual deformity cited in the articles, this is probably a technique best used when confronted with an extremely stiff foot or, better yet, multiple arthrodeses. The problem of recurrence is probably related to unidentified muscular imbalances preoperatively, such as the anterior tibialis or the toe flexors. These should be carefully evaluated preoperatively, then dealt with early to prevent plastic deformation of the foot post-osteotomy healing and frame removal.

In order to attain a more anatomic correction, but sidestep the potential vascular and wound healing issues of an acute correction, a few investigators used the Ilizarov frame to obtain gradual correction after soft tissue releases. They theorize that by decreasing the joint stiffness, the frame could achieve correction through the appropriate joints, without placing undue stress across physes or unintended joints.[88–90] Nakase and colleagues[90] performed complete subtalar releases (in the style of Simons[14]) prior to applying an Ilizarov frame for gradual correction for 6 recurrent clubfeet, with a mean patient age of 7.4 years. At a mean of 5.1 years, all the feet were reportedly plantigrade and parental satisfaction was high, despite 1 foot requiring further surgery for recurrence of adductus and 2 cases of spontaneous subtalar arthrodesis. A less favorable report was provided by Freedman and colleagues,[89] who described a group of patients with idiopathic and arthrogrypotic clubfeet who underwent similar treatment, at an average age of 5.7 years. Six of the 8 idiopathic clubfeet and all 4 of the arthrogrypotic clubfeet had a fair or poor outcome at an average 6.6 years' follow-up. The average time in frame was 62 days in Nakase and colleagues' study and 28 days in Freedman and colleagues', suggesting that time in frame after correction may have an impact on outcomes.

The earliest articles on the use of the Ilizarov frame for correction of neglected or relapsed clubfoot deformities published in English were by Grill, Franke, and colleagues.[75,76] Rather than perform osteotomies or soft tissue releases to facilitate correction with the external fixator, they relied on soft tissue distraction to gradually correct bony alignment. In their initial 1987 article, they described 4 idiopathic clubfeet (2 neglected and 2 relapsed) and 1 arthrogrypotic clubfoot, with an average age of 11 years. At an average 3.3 years' follow-up, all feet were found to be plantigrade, although only after further procedures in 3 feet. Stiffness of the subtalar and midtarsal joints was common.[75] In their 1990 follow-up article, 6 idiopathic and 4 arthrogrypotic clubfeet were included, all of which were plantigrade, and all participants were satisfied with the results at an average follow-up of 5 years, especially because they could now wear standard shoes.[76] Since those studies, there has been an expanding body of data in support of clubfoot treatment with the Ilizarov external fixator through soft tissue distraction. de la Huerta[91] had the only study limited to adults with neglected clubfeet (average age 27 years). When the 12 feet were reviewed 2 to 5 years after frame removal, all patients were satisfied with their feet, despite relapse of adductus in 25% and 1 patient requiring release of iatrogenic claw toes bilaterally.

In the article by Kocaoğlu and colleagues[78] on Ilizarov-treated clubfeet, 5 clubfeet were treated by soft tissue distraction alone at an average age of 7.4 years. One developed a recurrence after frame removal, but the other 4 remained plantigrade at an average 2-years' follow-up. The series by El-Mowafi and colleagues[83] featured 19 feet treated by soft tissue distraction at an average age of 10.5 years. At an average 5.6 years' follow-up, foot pressure measurements showed that only 3 of the 19 feet were not plantargrade, of which 2 feet underwent a repeat soft tissue distraction and none required soft tissue releases or osteotomies. In both these articles, patients were treated with either soft tissue distraction or osteotomies; those treated with soft tissue distraction overall had better outcomes than those patients treated with osteotomies.

Wallander and colleagues[92] treated 10 clubfeet with soft tissue distraction, at an average of 10 years of age. Their technique included gradual joint distraction punctuated by repeated returns to the operating room for frame adjustments to correct the varus and equinus until the deformity was fully corrected; 80% of the patients were satisfied, although 50% had equinus contractures and 60% experienced occasional pain at a follow-up median of 40 months. Hosny[93] treated 13 clubfeet with an average

age of 12 years. At an average of 15 months' postframe removal, 11 feet rated good and the other 2 were fair. Bradish and Noor[94] treated 17 relapsed clubfeet with soft tissue distraction, with a mean age of 7.8 years. At a mean of 3 years' follow-up, 13 feet had good or excellent outcomes; the 4 that were fair or poor had varying degrees of residual equinus, varus, supination, or adductus. Five of the "excellent" feet underwent planned split tibialis anterior tendon transfers 2 weeks after frame removal for preoperatively mobile but deformed feet. Prem and colleagues[95] had one of the longer follow-ups (mean of 6.9 years) on this topic—on 19 clubfeet with a mean age of 5 years. Using the International Clubfoot Study Group scoring system,[96] 14 feet rated good or excellent. Only 1 patient was dissatisfied due to a relapse, but the majority of the feet had ankle and subtalar joint stiffness. El Barbary and colleagues[97] had the largest series—66 neglected or relapsed clubfeet all treated with soft tissue distraction at a mean age of 8.5 years. At a mean follow-up of 40 months, despite a recurrence of forefoot adductus in 8 feet, all feet were plantigrade.

Lamm and colleagues[82] were among the first to describe marrying the concepts of the Ponseti method[1] with external fixator correction. They used the Taylor Spatial Frame, correcting internal rotation and varus in the first stage; then, a second program was run for equinus correction. They did not publish any patient data, however. Tripathy and colleagues[98] used an Ilizarov frame with a similar purpose, for 15 neglected or relapsed clubfeet with a mean age of 7.3 years. Cavus was corrected acutely during frame application by a percutaneous plantar fasciotomy; then the frame was used to first gradually correct the forefoot adductus, allowing the unfixated calcaneus to spontaneously roll into valgus. Once the foot was well corrected, a frame adjustment and Achilles tenotomy were performed for correction of equinus. Deformity correction was well achieved, transfiguring all the feet from Dimeglio grades[99] III and IV to grades I and II. The functional score at average 2.5 years, using the Laaveg and Ponseti rating system,[4] showed significant overall improvement from preoperative status, but only 5 feet scored good or excellent; the remaining 10 were fair or poor.

Similar to Tripathy and colleagues, Ferreira and colleagues[100,101] performed plantar fasciotomies and percutaneous Achilles tenotomies at the time of fixator application; 38 neglected clubfeet treated at an average 19 years of age were reviewed at an average of 58 months—30 feet had good results, but 8 had fair or poor results, and overall 50% of feet had at least mild recurrence that did not apparently affect function or satisfaction. Spontaneous ankylosis of the foot and ankle joints were observed in 74% of patients, and 24% of feet required arthrodeses of the midfoot or ankle to treat residual deformities or symptomatic arthritis. Refai and colleagues[102] also preformed plantar fascia releases, along with a release of the abductor hallucis muscle at the time of Ilizarov application. The investigators' unique contribution was a closed pinning of the talonavicular and calcaneocuboid joints in the corrected position at the time of frame removal; 19 feet were treated at an average age of 8 years, and at 4.5 years' average follow-up, 16 feet were plantigrade and pain-free.

The technique of using an external fixator for soft tissue distraction of the clubfoot seems to have many benefits, because it does not shorten the foot, and there is a limited risk of neurovascular compromise. The studies are difficult to interpret or extrapolate, as they use varying and noncomparable standards by which to rate outcomes, and they are all of short follow-up. In many studies, the majority of patients had not reached skeletal maturity at the time of final review.[92–95,97,102] Investigators noted several reoccurring complications, other than deformity recurrences and pin tract infections. Toe contractures and metatarsalphalangeal joint subluxations or dislocations occurred frequently.[75,76,78,91–94,97,100–102] Prevention is the best treatment, either using toe slings and physical therapy to maintain flexibility, or, my preference, prophylactically pinning the toes and attaching those pins to the forefoot ring to act as supplemental stabilization. Stiffness of the ankle or subtalar and/or midfoot joints was often noted,[75,76,91,95,100,101] although this may reflect more the initial deformity than response to treatment. A high rate of spontaneous ankylosis or arthritis, recorded by one group,[100,101] may reflect a lack of joint distraction during forced correction, which may place undue pressure on the articular cartilage, leading to breakdown and subsequent stiffness, degeneration, or ankylosis.

THE PONSETI METHOD FOR TREATING NEGLECTED OR RELAPSED CLUBFEET

Although Ponseti did not state an age limit beyond which his method would no longer be appropriate, his studies only included babies 6 months or younger at the start of treatment.[1,4,16,28] Recently, several international investigators began applying the method to older children. Göksan and colleagues[19] treated 134 feet under 1 year of age with the Ponseti method; 31% percent of the feet relapsed, requiring recasting in most cases; second relapses in 18 feet required tibialis anterior transfers. At a mean follow-up of 46 months, maintenance of correction was attained without joint releases in 97% of the feet. Relapses occurred in only 3% of brace compliant patients and 68% of noncompliant patients. Alves and colleagues,[17] in a study of 102 clubfeet, found that children between the ages 6 months and 2.5 years responded as well to the Ponseti method as those younger than 6 months. In none of the cases was a posteromedial release required. Hegazy and colleagues[20] reported on a cohort that had failed manipulative treatment elsewhere, aged 4 to 13 months. Only 1 of the 32 feet required a posteromedial release, the only unsatisfactory result in that series. In a Nepalese study of 260 neglected clubfeet of children ranging in age from 1 to 6 years, Spiegel and colleagues[22] found that only 37 (14%) required soft tissue releases. The child's age at the start of treatment did not have an impact on the number of casts needed or the ability to attain correction. Lourenço and Morcuende[103] had an even greater age range (1.2–9.0 years) for the 24 patients in their study of neglected clubfeet. The mean follow-up was 3.1 years. Equinus recurrence required correction in 15 patients, 7 of whom were treated with a repeat Achilles tenotomy, 8 with a posterior release; 16 of the 24 patients were rated as a good result. Khan and Kumar[21] prospectively studied children over 7 years of age with neglected clubfeet, reporting on 25 feet with at least 4 years' follow-up; 19 feet did well, with good flexibility at follow-up. Six feet (24%) relapsed, requiring posteromedial releases. The study that pushed the age boundary the most was the multicenter study by Nogueira and colleagues,[104] who corrected 83 clubfeet after relapses resulting from previous posteromedial releases. The age range was 7 months to 14 years, average 5 months. At an average follow-up of 45 months, 71 feet were plantargrade. One patient had no correction of his hindfoot varus after 10 casts, and a surgical exploration was positive for a subtalar synostosis. Of the 12 relapses, only 6 required surgery (tibialis anterior tendon transfer) and 3 of those also required lateral column shortening, plantar fasciotomy, and Achilles tendon lengthening. They found no relationship between outcomes scores and age.

SUMMARY AND AUTHOR'S PREFERENCES

Neglected and relapsed clubfeet are a challenge to treat. For mild and supple relapse, muscle rebalancing by way of a tibialis anterior tendon transfer may be successful, if the primary deformity is a dynamic supination/adductus/inversion. The foot should be corrected with serial casting first, and an Achilles tenotomy is often necessary. More-extensive soft tissue releases overall seem to have a high recurrence rate and are rarely the procedure of choice, particularly in the face of poor skin quality.

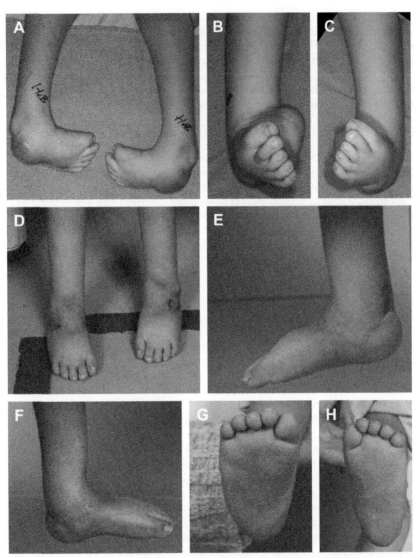

Fig. 1. A 3-year-old boy with bilateral neglected arthrogrypotic clubfeet. (*A*). Precasting anteroposterior view of both feet, oriented by ankle. (*B*) Precasting medial view of right foot, oriented by ankle. (*C*) Precasting medial view of left foot, oriented by ankle. (*D*) Anteroposterior standing view of bilateral feet after an initial percutaneous Achilles tenotomy, 9 Ponseti-style stretching casts, and a second precutaneous Achilles tenotomy for residual equinus, requiring 10 casts over 12 weeks. (*E*) Medial view of right foot, post-treatment. (*F*) Medial view of left foot, post-treatment. (*G*) Plantar surface of right foot, post-treatment. (*H*) Plantar surface of left foot, post-treatment.

Osteotomies along the midfoot (cuneiform-cuboid axis), the lateral column (Evans or Lichtblau), or calcaneus (Dwyer) are best suited for correction of specific isolated deformities (ie, adductus without supination or heel varus with a plantargrade forefoot) and probably should be delayed to as close to skeletal maturity as possible, to prevent further growth related deformity. Triple arthrodeses and talectomies should have a limited role in clubfoot treatment, especially the idiopathic deformity. Their use should be reserved for only the most extreme situations, where there are no resources available for other treatment options (serial casting or Ilizarov frames).

My practice is somewhat unique in that children with arthrogryposis multiplex congenita make up 75% of my clinical load and a large majority of the clubfoot deformities seen. I also see a large number of older children with neglected or relapsed clubfeet, in many cases adopted from abroad. I have not performed soft tissue releases on any of these children in 13 years. I began treating infant arthrogrypotic clubfeet with the Ponseti method, obtaining results better than those published for surgically treated arthrogryposis multiplex congenita clubfeet.[105] Initially, I treated the older children (over 4–5 years) with midfoot and calcaneal osteotomies and gradual correction with an Ilizarov frame. As casting results improved and the applicable age range expanded, Ilizarov treatment was reserved for children over 10 years of age. Several feet treated with osteotomies and Ilizarov frames developed stiff relapses and unintentional arthrodeses, which inspired the conversion to using the Ilizarov frame for soft tissue distraction in the style of Ponseti, in my practice. Then came the pivotal case of an 11-year-old girl with bilateral neglected arthrogrypotic clubfeet, where the cavus/adductus/supination was so severe that it was not possible to apply a frame medially to fixate the forefoot. Therefore, I performed preliminary Achilles tenotomies and applied 8 Ponseti casts. This corrected the foot well enough for frame placement, and the rest of the deformity was corrected by soft tissue distraction. The initial correction obtained by casting her feet, however, gave me confidence in later cases to continue casting these severe feet to ultimate correction, including in patients who were skeletally mature with neglected arthrogrypotic clubfeet. I have been treating all feet in this manner for the past 2 years (**Fig. 1**).

My treatment paradigm currently is to treat all clubfeet, regardless of age or previous treatment, with Ponseti casting, unless radiographs indicate bony synostosis from previous treatment. Occasionally, a percutaneous tenotomy is needed either initially or in midcasting, if the extreme equinus locks the calcaneus to the posterior tibia and restricts the ability of the calcaneus to roll into valgus. A second percutaneous tenotomy may be needed at the end of treatment to address residual equinus. Sometimes, toe flexor tenotomies are required initially as well, if there are severe flexion contractures. Postcorrection, the feet are carefully maintained at all times in ankle-foot orthoses, with straps to stretch the ankle into dorsiflexion at night. The Ilizarov frame is primarily used in cases of bony synostosis, with osteotomies across the cuneiform-cuboid axis and the posterior tuberosity of the calcaneus.

The tibialis anterior should be carefully assessed prior to surgery, because it is often the cause of relapses and has a high likelihood of potentiating yet another recurrence. A transfer of the tibialis anterior, after correction has been attained, can help prevent the problems inherent to an imbalanced foot.[5,19]

REFERENCES

1. Ponseti IV. Congenital clubfoot: fundamentals of treatment. New York: Oxford University Press Inc; 1996. p. 98.
2. Bensahel H, Catterall A, Dimeglio A. Practical applications in idiopathic clubfoot: a retrospective multicentric study in EPOS. J Pediatr Orthop 1990;10(2):186–8.
3. Morcuende JA, Dolan LA, Dietz FR, et al. Radical reduction in the rate of extensive corrective surgery for clubfoot using the Ponseti method. Pediatrics 2004; 113(2):376–80.

4. Laaveg SJ, Ponseti IV. Long-term results of treatment of congenital club foot. J Bone Joint Surg Am 1980;62(1):23–31.

5. Ponseti IV, Smoley EN. Congenital club foot: the results of treatment. J Bone Joint Surg Am 1963;45(2):261–75, 344.

6. Tarraf YN, Carroll NC. Analysis of the components of residual deformity in clubfeet presenting for reoperation. J Pediatr Orthop 1992;12(2):207–16.

7. Feldbrin Z, Gilai AN, Ezra E, et al. Muscle imbalance in the aetiology of idiopathic club foot. An electromyographic study. J Bone Joint Surg Br 1995; 77(4):596–601.

8. Zimny ML, Willig SJ, Roberts JM, et al. An electron microscopic study of the fascia from the medial and lateral sides of clubfoot. J Pediatr Orthop 1985; 5(5):577–81.

9. Fukuhara K, Schollmeier G, Uhthoff HK. The pathogenesis of club foot. A histomorphometric and immunohistochemical study of fetuses. J Bone Joint Surg Br 1994;76(3):450–7.

10. Khan AM, Ryan MG, Gruber MM, et al. Connective tissue structures in clubfoot: a morphologic study. J Pediatr Orthop 2001;21(6):708–12.

11. Thacker MM, Scher DM, Sala DA, et al. Use of the foot abduction orthosis following Ponseti casts: is it essential? J Pediatr Orthop 2005;25(2):225–8.

12. Turco VJ. Surgical correction of the resistant club foot. One-stage posteromedial release with internal fixation: a preliminary report. J Bone Joint Surg Am 1971; 53(3):477–97.

13. Turco VJ. Resistant congenital club foot–one-stage posteromedial release with internal fixation. A follow-up report of a fifteen-year experience. J Bone Joint Surg Am 1979;61(6A):805–14.

14. Simons GW. Complete subtalar release in club feet. Part I–A preliminary report. J Bone Joint Surg Am 1985;67(7):1044–55.

15. Simons GW. The complete subtalar release in clubfeet. Orthop Clin North Am 1987;18(4):667–88.

16. Cooper DM, Dietz FR. Treatment of idiopathic clubfoot. A thirty-year follow-up note. J Bone Joint Surg Am 1995;77(10):1477–89.

17. Alves C, Escalda C, Fernandes P, et al. Ponseti method: does age at the beginning of treatment make a difference? Clin Orthop Relat Res 2009;467(5):1271–7.

18. Bor N, Herzenberg JE, Frick SL. Ponseti management of clubfoot in older infants. Clin Orthop Relat Res 2006;444:224–8.

19. Göksan SB, Bursali A, Bilgili F, et al. Ponseti technique for the correction of idiopathic clubfeet presenting up to 1 year of age. A preliminary study in children with untreated or complex deformities. Arch Orthop Trauma Surg 2006;126(1): 15–21.

20. Hegazy M, Nasef NM, Abdel-Ghani H. Results of treatment of idiopathic clubfoot in older infants using the Ponseti method: a preliminary report. J Pediatr Orthop B 2009;18(2):76–8.

21. Khan SA, Kumar A. Ponseti's manipulation in neglected clubfoot in children more than 7 years of age: a prospective evaluation of 25 feet with long-term follow-up. J Pediatr Orthop B 2010;19(5):385–9.

22. Spiegel DA, Shrestha OP, Sitoula P, et al. Ponseti method for untreated idiopathic clubfeet in Nepalese patients from 1 to 6 years of age. Clin Orthop Relat Res 2009;467(5):1164–70.

23. Pirani S, Zeznik L, Hodges D. Magnetic resonance imaging study of the congenital clubfoot treated with the Ponseti method. J Pediatr Orthop 2001;21(6): 719–26.

24. Dobbs MB, Corley CL, Morcuende JA, et al. Late recurrence of clubfoot deformity: a 45-year followup. Clin Orthop Relat Res 2003;(411):188–92.
25. Salinas G, Chotigavanichaya C, Otsuka NY. A 30 year functional follow-up of a neglected congenital clubfoot in an adult: a case report. Foot Ankle Int 2000; 21(12):1037–9.
26. Garceau GJ. Anterior tibial tendon transposition in recurrent congenital clubfoot. J Bone Joint Surg Am 1940;22(4):932–6.
27. Garceau GJ, Palmer RM. Transfer of the anterior tibial tendon for recurrent club foot. A long-term follow-up. J Bone Joint Surg Am 1967;49(2):207–31.
28. Ponseti IV. Treatment of congenital club foot. J Bone Joint Surg Am 1992;74(3): 448–54.
29. Kuo KN, Hennigan SP, Hastings ME. Anterior tibial tendon transfer in residual dynamic clubfoot deformity. J Pediatr Orthop 2001;21(1):35–41.
30. Farsetti P, Caterini R, Mancini F, et al. Anterior tibial tendon transfer in relapsing congenital clubfoot: long-term follow-up study of two series treated with a different protocol. J Pediatr Orthop 2006;26(1):83–90.
31. Gartland JJ, Surgent RE. Posterior tibial transplant in the surgical treatment of recurrent clubfoot. Clin Orthop Relat Res 1972;84:66–70.
32. Park SS, Kim SW, Jung BS, et al. Selective soft-tissue release for recurrent or residual deformity after conservative treatment of idiopathic clubfoot. J Bone Joint Surg Br 2009;91(11):1526–30.
33. Bensahel H, Csukonyi Z, Desgrippes Y, et al. Surgery in residual clubfoot: one-stage medioposterior release "a la carte". J Pediatr Orthop 1987;7(2):145–8.
34. Bost FC, Schottstaedt ER, Larsen LJ. Plantar dissection. An operation to release the soft tissues in recurrent or recalcitrant talipes equinovarus. J Bone Joint Surg Am 1960;42(1):151–76.
35. Sherman FC, Westin GW. Plantar release in the correction of deformities of the foot in childhood. J Bone Joint Surg Am 1981;63(9):1382–9.
36. Khan MA, Chinoy MA. Treatment of severe and neglected clubfoot with a double zigzag incision: outcome of 21 feet in 15 patients followed up between 1 and 5 years. J Foot Ankle Surg 2006;45(3):177–81.
37. Reize C, Ulrich Exner G. Acute correction of severe neglected club feet using a circumferential incision. J Pediatr Orthop B 2007;16(3):213–5.
38. D'Souza H, Aroojis A, Yagnik MG. Rotation fasciocutaneous flap for neglected clubfoot: a new technique. J Pediatr Orthop 1998;18(3):319–22.
39. Purushothamdas S, Rayan F, Gayner A. Correction of neglected clubfoot deformity in children with Moebius syndrome. J Pediatr Orthop B 2009; 18(2):73–5.
40. Hassan FO, Jabaiti S, El tamimi T. Complete subtalar release for older children who had recurrent clubfoot deformity. Foot Ankle Surg 2010;16(1):38–44.
41. Bassett GS, Mazur KU, Sloan GM. Soft-tissue expander failure in severe equinovarus foot deformity. J Pediatr Orthop 1993;13(6):744–8.
42. Silver L, Grant AD, Atar D, et al. Use of tissue expansion in clubfoot surgery. Foot Ankle 1993;14(3):117–22.
43. Kuhns CA, Zeegen EN, Kono M, et al. Growth rates in skeletally immature feet after triple arthrodesis. J Pediatr Orthop 2003;23(4):488–92.
44. McCauley JC. Triple arthrodesis for congenital talipes equinovarus deformities. Clin Orthop Relat Res 1964;34:25–9.
45. Evans D. Treatment of the unreduced or 'relapsed' club foot in older children. Proc R Soc Med 1968;61(8):782–3.
46. Evans D. Relapsed club foot. J Bone Joint Surg 1961;43B:722–33.

47. Tayton K, Thompson P. Relapsing club feet. Late results of delayed operation. J Bone Joint Surg Br 1979;61-B(4):474–80.
48. Graham GP, Dent CM. Dillwyn Evans operation for relapsed club foot. Long-term results. J Bone Joint Surg Br 1992;74(3):445–8.
49. Lichtblau S. A medial and lateral release operation for club foot. A preliminary report. J Bone Joint Surg Am 1973;55(7):1377–84.
50. Mehrafshan M, Rampal V, Seringe R, et al. Recurrent club-foot deformity following previous soft-tissue release: mid-term outcome after revision surgery. J Bone Joint Surg Br 2009;91(7):949–54.
51. Hofmann AA, Constine RM, McBride GG, et al. Osteotomy of the first cuneiform as treatment of residual adduction of the fore part of the foot in club foot. J Bone Joint Surg Am 1984;66(7):985–90.
52. McHale KA, Lenhart MK. Treatment of residual clubfoot deformity–the "bean-shaped" foot–by opening wedge medial cuneiform osteotomy and closing wedge cuboid osteotomy. Clinical review and cadaver correlations. J Pediatr Orthop 1991;11(3):374–81.
53. Lourenco AF, Dias LS, Zoellick DM, et al. Treatment of residual adduction deformity in clubfoot: the double osteotomy. J Pediatr Orthop 2001;21(6):713–8.
54. Pohl M, Nicol RO. Transcuneiform and opening wedge medial cuneiform osteotomy with closing wedge cuboid osteotomy in relapsed clubfoot. J Pediatr Orthop 2003;23(1):70–3.
55. Kose N, Gunal I, Gokturk E, et al. Treatment of severe residual clubfoot deformity by trans-midtarsal osteotomy. J Pediatr Orthop B 1999;8(4):251–6.
56. Mahadev A, Munajat I, Mansor A, et al. Combined lateral and transcuneiform without medial osteotomy for residual clubfoot for children. Clin Orthop Relat Res 2009;467(5):1319–25.
57. Davidson RS. Clubfoot salvage: a review of the past decade's contributions. J Pediatr Orthop 2003;23(3):410–8.
58. Farsetti P, De Maio F, Russolillo L, et al. CT study on the effect of different treatment protocols for clubfoot pathology. Clin Orthop Relat Res 2009;467(5):1243–9.
59. Dwyer FC. Treatment of the relapsed club foot. Proc R Soc Med 1968;61(8):783.
60. Dwyer FC. The treatment of relapsed club foot by insertion of a wedge into the calcaneum. J Bone Joint Surg 1963;45B:67–75.
61. Kumar PN, Laing PW, Klenerman L. Medial calcaneal osteotomy for relapsed equinovarus deformity. Long-term study of the results of Frederick Dwyer. J Bone Joint Surg Br 1993;75(6):967–71.
62. Lundberg BJ. Early Dwyer operation in talipes equinovarus. Clin Orthop Relat Res 1981;(154):223–7.
63. Souchet P, Ilharreborde B, Fitoussi F, et al. Calcaneal derotation osteotomy for clubfoot revision surgery. J Pediatr Orthop B 2007;16(3):209–13.
64. Napiontek M, Nazar J. Tibial osteotomy as a salvage procedure in the treatment of congenital talipes equinovarus. J Pediatr Orthop 1994;14(6):763–7.
65. Farsetti P, Dragoni M, Ippolito E. Tibiofibular torsion in congenital clubfoot. J Pediatr Orthop B 2012;21(1):47–51.
66. el-Tayeby HM. The neglected clubfoot: a salvage procedure. J Foot Ankle Surg 1998;37(6):501–9.
67. Abrams RC. Relapsed club foot. The early results of an evaluation of Dillwyn Evans' operation. J Bone Joint Surg Am 1969;51(2):270–82.
68. Herold HZ, Torok G. Surgical correction of neglected club foot in the older child and adult. J Bone Joint Surg Am 1973;55(7):1385–95.

69. Lui TH. Case report: correction of neglected club foot deformity by arthroscopic assisted triple arthrodesis. Arch Orthop Trauma Surg 2010;130(8):1007–11.
70. Sobel E, Giorgini R, Velez Z. Surgical correction of adult neglected clubfoot: three case histories. J Foot Ankle Surg 1996;35(1):27–38.
71. Joseph TN, Myerson MS. Use of talectomy in modern foot and ankle surgery. Foot Ankle Clin 2004;9:775–85.
72. Cooper RR, Capello W. Talectomy. A long-term follow-up evaluation. Clin Orthop Relat Res 1985;(201):32–5.
73. Legaspi J, Li YH, Chow W, et al. Talectomy in patients with recurrent deformity in club foot. A long-term follow-up study. J Bone Joint Surg Br 2001;83(3):384–7.
74. Mirzayan R, Early SD, Matthys GA, et al. Single-stage talectomy and tibiocalcaneal arthrodesis as a salvage of severe, rigid equinovarus deformity. Foot Ankle Int 2001;22(3):209–13.
75. Grill F, Franke J. The Ilizarov distractor for the correction of relapsed or neglected clubfoot. J Bone Joint Surg Br 1987;69(4):593–7.
76. Franke J, Grill F, Hein G, et al. Correction of clubfoot relapse using Ilizarov's apparatus in children 8-15 years old. Arch Orthop Trauma Surg 1990;110(1): 33–7.
77. Grant AD, Atar D, Lehman WB. The Ilizarov technique in correction of complex foot deformities. Clin Orthop Relat Res 1992;(280):94–103.
78. Kocaoğlu M, Eralp L, Atalar AC, et al. Correction of complex foot deformities using the Ilizarov external fixator. J Foot Ankle Surg 2002;41(1):30–9.
79. Paley D. The correction of complex foot deformities using Ilizarov's distraction osteotomies. Clin Orthop Relat Res 1993;(293):97–111.
80. Dhar S. Ilizarov external fixation in the correction of severe pediatric foot and ankle deformities. Foot Ankle Clin 2010;15(2):265–85.
81. Koutsogiannis E. Treatment of mobile flat foot by displacement osteotomy of the calcaneus. J Bone Joint Surg Br 1971;53(1):96–100.
82. Lamm BM, Standard SC, Galley IJ, et al. External fixation for the foot and ankle in children. Clin Podiatr Med Surg 2006;23(1):137–66, ix.
83. El-Mowafi H, El-Alfy B, Refai M. Functional outcome of salvage of residual and recurrent deformities of clubfoot with Ilizarov technique. Foot Ankle Surg 2009; 15(1):3–6.
84. Segev E, Ezra E, Yaniv M, et al. V osteotomy and Ilizarov technique for residual idiopathic or neurogenic clubfeet. J Orthop Surg (Hong Kong) 2008;16(2): 215–9.
85. Utukuri MM, Ramachandran M, Hartley J, et al. Patient-based outcomes after Ilizarov surgery in resistant clubfeet. J Pediatr Orthop B 2006;15(4):278–84.
86. Eidelman M, Keren Y, Katzman A. Correction of residual clubfoot deformities in older children using the Taylor spatial butt frame and midfoot Gigli saw osteotomy. J Pediatr Orthop 2012;32(5):527–33.
87. Burns JK, Sullivan R. Correction of severe residual clubfoot deformity in adolescents with the Ilizarov technique. Foot Ankle Clin 2004;9(3):571–82, ix.
88. Correll J, Forth A. Correction of severe clubfoot by the Ilizarov method. Foot Ankle Surg 1996;2:27–32.
89. Freedman JA, Watts H, Otsuka NY. The Ilizarov method for the treatment of resistant clubfoot: is it an effective solution? J Pediatr Orthop 2006;26(4): 432–7.
90. Nakase T, Yasui N, Ohzono K, et al. Treatment of relapsed idiopathic clubfoot by complete subtalar release combined with the Ilizarov method. J Foot Ankle Surg 2006;45(5):337–41.

91. de la Huerta F. Correction of the neglected clubfoot by the Ilizarov method. Clin Orthop Relat Res 1994;(301):89–93.
92. Wallander H, Hansson G, Tjernstrom B. Correction of persistent clubfoot deformities with the Ilizarov external fixator. Experience in 10 previously operated feet followed for 2–5 years. Acta Orthop Scand 1996;67(3):283–7.
93. Hosny GA. Correction of foot deformities by the Ilizarov method without corrective osteotomies or soft tissue release. J Pediatr Orthop B 2002;11(2):121–8.
94. Bradish CF, Noor S. The Ilizarov method in the management of relapsed club feet. J Bone Joint Surg Br 2000;82(3):387–91.
95. Prem H, Zenios M, Farrell R, et al. Soft tissue Ilizarov correction of congenital talipes equinovarus–5 to 10 years postsurgery. J Pediatr Orthop 2007;27(2): 220–4.
96. Bensahela H, Kuo K, Duhaime M, et al. Outcome evaluation of the treatment of clubfoot: the international language of clubfoot. J Pediatr Orthop B 2003;12(4): 269–71.
97. El Barbary H, Abdel Ghani H, Hegazy M. Correction of relapsed or neglected clubfoot using a simple Ilizarov frame. Int Orthop 2004;28(3):183–6.
98. Tripathy SK, Saini R, Sudes P, et al. Application of the Ponseti principle for deformity correction in neglected and relapsed clubfoot using the Ilizarov fixator. J Pediatr Orthop B 2011;20(1):26–32.
99. Dimeglio A, Bensahel H, Souchet P, et al. Classification of clubfoot. J Pediatr Orthop B 1995;4(2):129–36.
100. Ferreira RC, Costa MT. Recurrent clubfoot–approach and treatment with external fixation. Foot Ankle Clin 2009;14(3):435–45.
101. Ferreira RC, Costo MT, Frizzo GG, et al. Correction of neglected clubfoot using the Ilizarov external fixator. Foot Ankle Int 2006;27(4):266–73.
102. Refai MA, Song SH, Song HR. Does short-term application of an Ilizarov frame with transfixion pins correct relapsed clubfoot in children? Clin Orthop Relat Res 2012;470(7):1992–9.
103. Lourenço AF, Morcuende JA. Correction of neglected idiopathic club foot by the Ponseti method. J Bone Joint Surg Br 2007;89(3):378–81.
104. Nogueira MP, Ey Batlle AM, Alves CG. Is it possible to treat recurrent clubfoot with the Ponseti technique after posteromedial release?: a preliminary study. Clin Orthop Relat Res 2009;467(5):1298–305.
105. van Bosse HJ, Marangoz S, Lehman WB, et al. Correction of arthrogrypotic clubfoot with a modified Ponseti technique. Clin Orthop Relat Res 2009; 467(5):1283–93.

The Intoeing Child
Etiology, Prognosis, and Current Treatment Options

Edwin Harris, DPM, FACFAS[a,b,]*

KEYWORDS

- Intoeing • Adducted gait • Hallux varus • Metatarsus adductus
- Talipes equinovarus • Pes cavus • Internal tibial torsion • Anteversion

KEY POINTS

- Intoeing is a common entrance complaint in infants, toddlers, and young children. Intoeing is best defined as internal rotation of the long axis of the foot to the line of progression.
- Intoeing may be caused by primary deformities within the foot, issues with tibial torsion, and femoral antetorsion (anteversion).
- Problems within the foot include hallux varus, metatarsus adductus, talipes equinovarus, and pes cavus. Each of these has specific treatments available.
- Management of tibial torsion is controversial, but not all cases spontaneously correct.
- Treatment must be individualized, and the risks and complications weighed against the predictable morbidity of intoeing.

INTRODUCTION

Parents understandably have worries about real and perceived imperfections in their children. Gait disturbances head the list, and intoeing is the most common concern. Consequently, physicians dealing with gait issues in infants and children must be thoroughly familiar with the causes, natural history, prognosis, goals, objectives, and limitations of treatment so that intoeing can be put into its proper perspective and managed effectively and realistically. From the physician's standpoint, one important question must be answered before embarking on evaluation and treatment. Considering that intoeing generates considerable caregiver angst and results in call for consultation, do intoeing children benefit medically from referral?[1] One study attempted to address this question by reviewing 202 referred patients. The majority of diagnoses were increased femoral anteversion (antetorsion) and internal tibial torsion. None of these patients required surgery, and 86% were discharged after the first visit. No significant abnormality was identified in 14% of the study population. Management and outcomes for these children were not affected by referral to the orthopedic clinic.[2]

[a] Department of Orthopaedics and Rehabilitation, Loyola University Chicago, Stritch School of Medicine, 2160 South First Avenue, Maywood, Illinois; [b] Private Practice, 10540 West Cermak Road, Westchester, IL 60154, USA
* Corresponding author. 10540 West Cermak Road, Westchester, IL 60154, USA.
E-mail address: Eharrisdpm@AOL.com

Clin Podiatr Med Surg 30 (2013) 531–565
http://dx.doi.org/10.1016/j.cpm.2013.07.002
0891-8422/13/$ – see front matter © 2013 Elsevier Inc. All rights reserved.

This finding highlights the problem in dealing with femoral antetorsion and tibial torsion. This attitude of frustration should not be extended to managing the treatable disorders such as talipes equinovarus, pes cavus, hallux varus, and metatarsus adductus.

DEFINING INTOEING

By definition, an intoeing gait pattern is unilateral or bilateral internal rotation of the long axis of the foot to the line of progression (the direction in which the child is moving). This process results in an internal foot progression angle and is regarded as an abnormality. Clarifying the issue, intoeing is not a diagnosis but is a clinical symptom of a more specific anatomic or functional diagnosis. The first step in successful management of intoeing is to identify the specific cause. In broad terms the underlying etiology may be a movement disorder, a static skeletal disorder, or combination of both.

OVERVIEW OF MANAGEMENT

Correct management of intoeing hinges on understanding the cause and subsequently the natural history of the intoeing.[3] Even the causes of the various types of rotational abnormalities are open to question. Are they in utero positioning problems, inherited issues, or arrests in development?[4] This aspect is especially true for the deformities within the foot.[5,6] In an attempt to address the in utero effect on limb development, one study was undertaken to assess the possible increased incidence of orthopedic deformities occurring in triplet pregnancies. The investigators found that only torticollis was increased in triplet pregnancies when compared with single births.[7]

The long-term repercussions for adult life must also be considered before attempts at management of intoeing are made. If there is no predictable long-term harm for most of these patients, this demands the evaluation of the risk-benefit ratio of therapy before considering invasive procedures. It also necessitates careful examination of the potential sites of intoeing.[8] One might question whether this concept of negativism should carry over to the easily treatable deformities in the foot, because they are known to have long-term consequences in adulthood, and are easily and successfully treated in infancy and early childhood.

The orthopedic literature generally considers the major causes of intoeing to be metatarsus adductus, tibial torsion, and femoral anteversion (antetorsion).[3,4,8–14] As far as foot deformities are concerned, the other treatable foot issues such as talipes equinovarus and pes cavus are not usually included. The absence of metatarsus adductus from the list of foot deformities may reflect the common belief that it either spontaneously corrects or is inconsequential. Movement disorder caused by neurologic dysfunction should also be added to the list of the causes of intoeing.

Because intoeing is a symptom and not an etiology, there may be several pathologic processes operating simultaneously. Neurologically abnormal children may intoe as the result of a primary movement disorder. Hemiplegics and diplegics intoe as the result of muscle imbalance. Usually the underlying central nervous system abnormality is known at the time of gait workup. However, on occasion, intoeing may be the symptom that leads to the diagnosis of neurologic dysfunction. With time, neurologic dysfunction causes permanent skeletal change that perpetuates the intoeing gait. In turn, this leads to further skeletal abnormality.

In the neurologically normal child, intoeing is usually caused by single or combinations of skeletal abnormality, which include abnormalities within the foot itself, in the tibiofibular segment, and in the relationship between the proximal and distal aspects of the femur[14]; abnormal position of the femoral head in the acetabulum; and abnormalities in the acetabulum itself.

Age at Onset of Symptoms

Causes of intoeing often can be anticipated based on the child's age at the onset of symptoms.[15] Deformities within the foot, such as metatarsus adductus, hallux varus, talipes equinovarus, and pes cavus, are all capable of producing an intoeing gait if they persist. However, these are very apparent in early infancy even on casual inspection. For this reason, most of these issues are identified and treated before the child begins to walk. Intoeing beginning between the ages of 1 and 2 years is most commonly caused by internal tibial torsion. Femoral anteversion (femoral antetorsion) is the most common reason for intoeing after the age of 2 years. One study suggests that tibial torsion is the most common cause for intoeing in children younger than 5, and beyond the age of 5 years the most common cause is femoral antetorsion. The 2 deformities often occur in combination.[16]

Identification of Cause

Determining the cause or causes of internal-rotation gait abnormalities requires careful examination of each of the 3 major areas of the anatomy that are known to produce intoeing. This concept led Staheli to coin the term "torsional profile."[17,18] This profile is composed of the foot-progression angle, internal and external rotation of the hip measured in the prone position, the thigh-foot angle, the transmalleolar axis measured in the prone knee-flexed position, and the foot shape.

INTOEING CAUSED BY PROBLEMS IN THE FOOT

Static deformities in the foot produce intoeing independent of any muscle imbalance, and include hallux varus, metatarsus adductus, talipes equinovarus, and various forms of cavoid disorder.

Hallux Varus

Hallux varus is defined as medial deviation of the longitudinal axis of the first proximal phalanx from the longitudinal axis of the first metatarsal. The result is adduction of the hallux. This definition presumes that the forefoot and rearfoot are otherwise normal, and the pathologic anatomy is adduction of the hallux independent of any other deformity (**Fig. 1**).

Etiology

Most hallux varus is due to either abnormal insertion of the abductor hallucis tendon or some degree of contracture of the muscle. This condition may be idiopathic, or may be a consequence after successful correction of metatarsus adductus or talipes equinovarus. The distance from origin to insertion of the abductor hallucis muscle becomes greater when the forefoot-adduction component of metatarsus adductus and talipes equinovarus is corrected.

Hallux varus may also be caused by developmental errors in the formation of the first ray. There may be complete or incomplete duplications of all or part of the first ray in the form of tibial polydactyly (**Fig. 2**). Recognizable bony segments may be identified on imaging, or there may only be fibrous tissue vestiges.

Clinical appearance

The hallux is deviated in a medial direction. The medial border of the foot proximal to the metatarsophalangeal joints is straight and does not show any medial concavity. This clinical finding helps distinguish hallux varus from metatarsus adductus (**Fig. 3**). The abnormal course of the abductor hallucis can frequently be palpated directly through the skin, and the examiner may notice that the tendon rides higher along

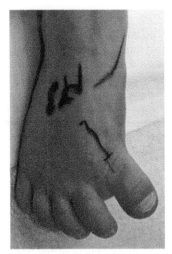

Fig. 1. There is adduction of the hallux, but the medial border of the foot proximal to the metatarsophalangeal joint is straight. There is no adduction of the first metatarsal.

the medial side of the first metatarsophalangeal joint instead of plantar. If contracture is present, it can be felt through the skin (**Fig. 4**).

Radiographs are critical for both diagnosis and treatment planning. Radiographs may demonstrate an adaptive change in the position of the articular surface of the first

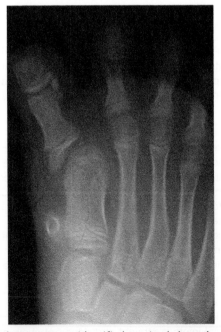

Fig. 2. There is an extra bony segment identified proximal along the medial first metatarsal. The medial base of the first proximal phalanx is anomalous, and there are several small bony fragments lateral to the interphalangeal joint in this child who had incomplete formation of an extra tibial ray. The first metatarsal is abnormally short.

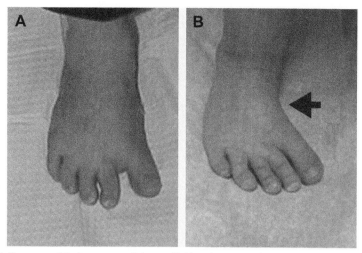

Fig. 3. Hallux varus (*A*) shows a straight medial border up to the metatarsophalangeal joint and an adducted hallux. Metatarsus adductus (*B*) shows a medial concavity with the apex at the first cuneiform (*arrow*).

metatarsal head in older children (**Fig. 5**), help distinguish hallux varus from metatarsus adductus (**Fig. 6**), and also identify the various forms of polydactyly.

Treatment

Hallux varus may be seen in otherwise normal infants and young children. In the absence of any other forefoot deformity, it is most probably the result either of

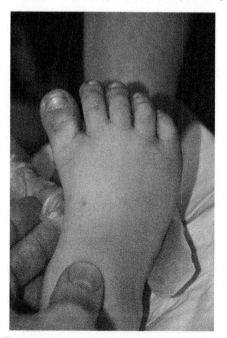

Fig. 4. The abductor hallucis tendon is contracted and can be palpated medially through the skin. When the examiner places pressure on it, the hallux adducts.

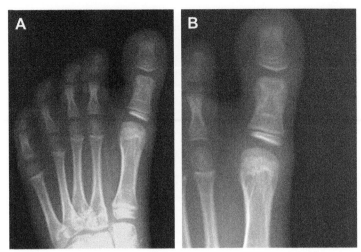

Fig. 5. (*A, B*) The head of the first metatarsal has developed change over time in this child with hallux varus. The proximal articular set angle has reversed.

abnormal insertion of the abductor hallucis or some form of contracture of the muscle. There is a possibility of spontaneous correction, and the problem may resolve without any treatment at all. If it is going to do so, this will happen before age 2 years. After that time, spontaneous correction is unlikely. The problem then becomes a surgical issue.

There are two surgical approaches. In the first, the abductor hallucis tendon can be sectioned through a small incision on the plantar and medial aspect of the distal first metatarsal. The tendon and distal fascia are delivered into the incision and simply cut. This approach is referred to as the Lichtblau procedure.[19] This author regards this

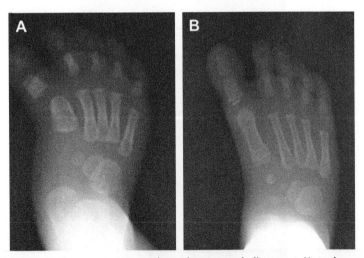

Fig. 6. Hallux varus shows a near normal tarsal-metatarsal alignment. Note the anomalous first metatarsal (*A*). Metatarsus adductus shows a deep concavity on the medial side of the foot with its apex at the first metatarsal base and first cuneiform. The lateral border of the foot is convex with its apex at the fifth metatarsal base (*B*).

procedure as palliative because there is a possibility that the tendon will regain continuity with the muscle, resulting in resumption of its abnormal activity. It should be reserved for those cases not suitable for more invasive surgery. In the second technique, the abductor hallucis tendon is transferred from its abnormal distal insertion to a better location at the medial portion of the flexor hallucis brevis just proximal to the tibial sesamoid. This technique is more technically demanding. The tendon is approached through a dorsomedial bunion-type incision running from the mid-proximal phalanx well proximal to the metatarsal head. As the incision is deepened, the muscle belly and tendon of abductor hallucis are visualized. The tendon is traced distally as far as possible and is released from the medial proximal phalanx. On occasion, the tendon and muscle may inadvertently be retracted with the skin, and the surgeon will have to explore the area carefully to find it. The fascia overlying the abductor hallucis is intimately fixated to the skin, and must be dissected free to fully mobilize the muscle and tendon. In most cases, there is a fibrous investiture surrounding the tendon as it passes over the medial portion of the metatarsophalangeal joint. It is important to carefully release this structure to allow the proximal phalanx to abduct on the metatarsal head. This goal is accomplished through several vertical incisions, taking care not to open the metatarsophalangeal joint capsule or injure the physis of the proximal phalanx.

There are several other issues to be surgically addressed. If hallux varus is a component of tibial (preaxial) polydactyly, there may be a fibrous vestige representing an incompletely formed medial ray; this is identified on surgical dissection and the abnormal tissue is excised.

Longitudinal epiphyseal bracket of the first metatarsal or the proximal phalanx can be a complicating factor of tibial polydactyly. In this lesion, the epiphyseal plate brackets the diaphysis and runs continuously along the medial side, which tethers the structure, causing shortening and varus angular deformity. The abnormal bracket can be excised. It is necessary to put either fat or methyl methacrylate into the resection site to prevent the bony bridge from reestablishing itself **(Fig. 7)**.[20,21]

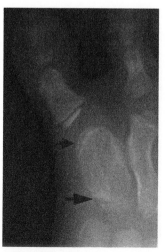

Fig. 7. The longitudinal epiphyseal bracket can be identified by the wraparound appearance of the epiphysis that extends from the base around the head of the metatarsal (*arrows*).

Metastarsus Adductus

Metatarsus adductus is a forefoot deformity based at the tarsometatarsal articulations. The first metatarsal is anatomically normal, but the first cuneiform is angulated or wedged distally with the apex directed medially; this adducts a structurally normal first metatarsal. The proximal lesser metatarsal shafts are angled in a medial direction just distal to their bases, which results in adduction of the metatarsal shafts with respect to the tarsus (**Fig. 8**). To explain another possible variant, Bleck introduced adduction of the talar neck as an additional potential cause.[9]

Metatarsus adductus is a generic term that includes pure transverse-plane adduction of the metatarsals, adduction and varus forms, and pure varus. It can also be classified by its resistance to passive overcorrection into rigid and flexible forms. Rigid deformities cannot be manually overcorrected, whereas flexible deformities are easily corrected with manual manipulation. Surprisingly, in the nonoperative management of metatarsus adductus by serial casting, it is the flexible deformity that has the poorest overall prognosis for successful reduction, as well as a much higher incidence of recurrence.

Etiology

The exact cause of metatarsus adductus is unknown. It can be unilateral or bilateral, and many cases are presumed to be caused by abnormal positioning in utero. However, there are numerous instances of multiple siblings and other first- and second-degree relatives who have metatarsus adductus, which suggests that there may be an hereditary component in at least some of the cases.

Clinical appearance

To qualify as metatarsus adductus, the rearfoot must be normal or minimally pronated. Any inversion of the rearfoot, forefoot plantarflexion, or any equinus of the ankle reclassifies the deformity into talipes equinovarus or pes cavus categories.

Most cases show the forefoot deviated purely transversely into adduction. This deviation produces a medial concavity of the foot with the apex of the deformity at the first metatarsal-first cuneiform area. On the lateral side of the foot, there is a convexity

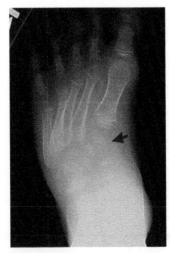

Fig. 8. Metatarsus adductus. The first metatarsal is normal in its shape. The first cuneiform is oblique distally (*arrow*). The lesser metatarsals are angled medially from a point just distal to the tarsometatarsal articulations.

with the apex at the base of the fifth metatarsal (**Fig. 9**). Less frequently, there is an adductovarus deformity with the forefoot both adducted and rotated into some degree of forefoot supination. Adductovarus forefoot deformity in association with a severely pronated rearfoot is better classified as skewfoot, and is not regarded as simple metatarsus adductus (**Fig. 10**).

Treatment

Treatment of metatarsus adductus is based on the age of the patient. Serial casting is the gold standard with which all other methods of treatment are compared. Casting takes advantage of the bioplasticity of the foot because most of the skeleton at the tarsometatarsal junctions is still cartilage. With the exception of the first metatarsal base, there are no epiphyseal plates in this area. Carefully molded casts abduct the metatarsals on the midfoot, and modify the shape of the metatarsal bases through the principles of cartilage remodeling in response to the forces applied. This procedure is possible up until the age of 24 to 30 months. At that point, there is an insufficient amount of cartilage remaining for this technique to work. Ideally, closed reduction of metatarsus adductus should begin at around 3 to 6 months of age. Although success is possible past the age of 1 year, there are some logistic problems that make this form of therapy difficult. The most important of these is that the child is now walking. It is difficult to maintain integrity of the casts in this age group because of weight bearing. Because of body weight and activity, there are also problems with skin tolerance. Bars have no place in the management of metatarsus adductus. Splints and abducting shoes generally are not reliable for the initial management of this disorder.

Surgical management of metatarsus adductus is salvage, for which two types of procedures are used. The first is tarsometatarsal release and serial casting, which was popularized as the Heyman-Herndon-Strong procedure.[22] It has fallen out of favor because of the development of arthrosis at the tarsometatarsal joint surfaces. In addition, some of the children develop plantarflexion of the forefoot against the rearfoot. For the procedure to succeed, the surgeon must perform an osteotomy of the second metatarsal base to mobilize all of the other metatarsals (**Fig. 11**).

The other procedures for metatarsus adductus involve osteotomy of the proximal metatarsals. A discussion of the various forms of osteotomy and their fixation techniques is beyond the scope of this article.

Opening wedge osteotomy of the 3 cuneiforms and closing osteotomy of the cuboid has also been proposed. This technique is commonly used for the management of forefoot adductus in talipes equinovarus. In metatarsus adductus, this procedure

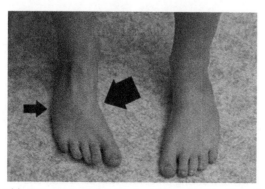

Fig. 9. Metatarsus adductus, more pronounced on the right side. Note the medial concavity (*large arrow*) and the lateral convexity with the apex at the fifth metatarsal (*small arrow*).

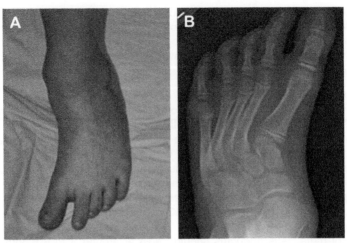

Fig. 10. (*A*) Skewfoot clinically resembles metatarsus adductus. (*B*) The radiograph shows severe adductus deformity of the metatarsals and an extremely wide talocalcaneal angle, with most of the talar head uncovered medially.

takes place proximal to the location of the true deformity and is not useful for this condition (**Fig. 12**).

Skewfoot Early recognition of skewfoot deformity is critical. It is unlikely to respond to nonoperative measures, and should not be confused with simple metatarsus adductus.[23–25] In most cases, the forefoot adductovarus is very severe, and the degree of peritalar subluxation requires at least lateral column lengthening.

Talipes Equinovarus

Talipes equinovarus results in an adducted foot. It is also characterized by heel varus and both forefoot and ankle equinus components. Older children with mild or

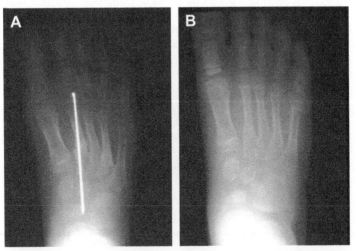

Fig. 11. (*A*) Heyman-Herndon-Strong procedure with osteotomy and fixation of the second metatarsal for metatarsus adductus. (*B*) When healed, the second metatarsal osteotomy totally remodels.

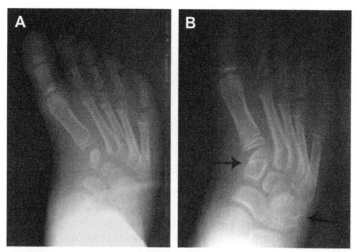

Fig. 12. (A) Preoperative radiograph of severe metatarsus adductus. (B) Postoperative radiograph of the same patient following open up osteotomy of the first cuneiform and closing osteotomy of the cuboid. There is virtually no improvement because the osteotomies (*arrows*) are done at a level far proximal to the apex of the true deformity.

uncorrected deformity will intoe, but almost always the other 2 components are sufficiently recognizable to make the correct diagnosis (**Fig. 13**).

Talipes equinovarus is not a pure diagnosis. Using the classification of Thompson and Simons,[26] 4 broad forms of this deformity can be recognized: the idiopathic variety, the postural (positional) type, the teratologic variations, and syndromic forms. Ponseti and colleagues[27] discussed another form of talipes equinovarus that they called complex talipes equinovarus. This condition is characterized by plantarflexion of both the medial and lateral columns, and is often associated with a short foot (**Fig. 14**).

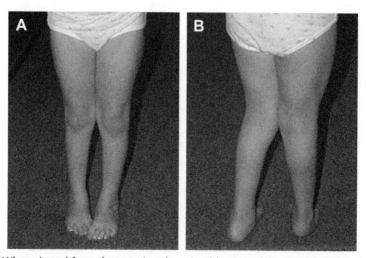

Fig. 13. When viewed from the anterior, there is adduction of the right foot (A). Note also the large dimpled area over the sinus tarsi of both feet characteristic of idiopathic talipes equinovarus. When viewed from the posterior, the right heel is inverted (B).

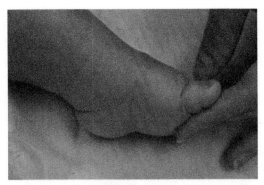

Fig. 14. The complex variation of talipes equinovarus as described by Ponseti.

Idiopathic talipes equinovarus accounts for the largest percentage of cases. It is better to regard even this type as a symptom complex rather than a specific disease, because there may be several causes producing similar lesions. There have been some studies suggesting that some cases are caused by a primary myopathy and others suggesting that there is some form of common peroneal nerve dysfunction.

Like the idiopathic form, the postural or positional type may have several potential causes. Most are thought to be the result of in utero molding, and they respond rapidly to manipulative treatment. However, some are the result of muscle imbalance, and either show a poor response to manipulative treatment or rapidly recur.

The teratogenic variety is associated with other orthopedic conditions such as myelomeningocele and various forms of arthrogryposis (**Fig. 15**).

The syndromic variations are associated with other clinical entities in which talipes equinovarus is an occasional or regularly occurring feature. These disorders include such aspects as chromosomal deletions, Larsen syndrome, fetal varicella sequence, clinically relevant occult spina bifida, myotonic dystrophy, and VACTERL association.

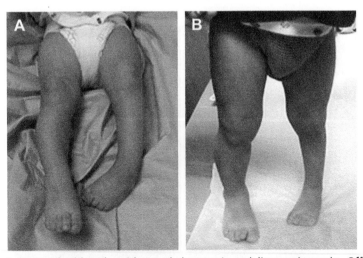

Fig. 15. A 27-month-old male with sacral dysgenesis and lipomeningocele. Off weight bearing, note the adductovarus deformity of the foot as well as tibial torsion (*A*). On weight bearing, the deformity persists. Note also the small transverse diameter of the left calf in comparison with the right (*B*).

Excessive internal rotation of the hips in infants with talipes equinovarus may be an overlooked explanation for internal gait abnormalities when these infants begin to walk,[28] and this most likely implicates femoral antetorsion as a comorbidity. Internal tibial torsion is occasionally seen with talipes equinovarus. It had erroneously been considered the fourth component of talipes equinovarus, but in fact is very uncommonly associated with talipes equinovarus (see **Fig. 15**). These observations drive home the point that internal rotation of the whole lower extremity can be a summation of abnormality in 2 or possibly 3 anatomic areas.

Etiology

Because talipes equinovarus is an anatomic deformity and not a specific disease, there are multiple potential causes. Histopathology of muscle showing fiber size and type disproportion has been identified by some investigators and discounted by others.[29–31] Some infants have abnormal electrodiagnostic studies and other investigations that implicate a neurologic involvement of the common peroneal nerve, especially in those clubfeet that recur.[32–34] Spinal cord abnormalities have also been reported.[35] The genetic component must not be overlooked. The incidence is roughly 2.5 in 1000 with a male/female ratio of approximately 2:1. One child with talipes equinovarus significantly increases the likelihood of subsequent siblings or other family members developing the same problem.

Clinical appearance

The neonatal appearance is very typical. The forefoot is adducted and the medial column is plantarflexed, which produces a cavoid appearance on the medial side of the foot. The peritalar area is supinated so that the navicular is on the inferior and medial portion of the talar head. The ankle is in equinus (**Fig. 16**).

In toddlers and older children with persisting or untreated deformity, the foot changes shape according to stresses placed on it through use. Almost always, it is internally rotated while maintaining the heel varus and the ankle equinus. The forefoot often develops a supination deformity.

Treatment

The worldwide acceptance of the Ponseti technique for closed reduction of talipes equinovarus has literally changed the prognosis and outcome for this deformity. Before that time, clinical management comprised initial casting followed by radical surgery that succeeded in producing a plantigrade foot. Unfortunately, many of the

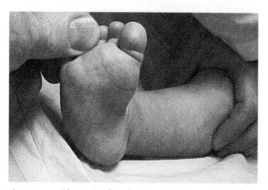

Fig. 16. Talipes equinovarus. There is forefoot adduction with first metatarsal plantar flexion, an inverted heel, and ankle in equinus.

feet became stiff and had secondary rearfoot deformities that negatively affected quality of life (**Fig. 17**).

Although an in-depth discussion of the Ponseti method is beyond the scope of this article, the procedure is briefly outlined. The earlier the child is treated, the better the results. However, it is possible to treat older infants, toddlers, and even young children with this technique. Above-the-knee casting is absolutely necessary, and most experienced surgeons still prefer plaster of Paris because it is superbly moldable. Casts are applied with an experienced assistant rolling the plaster of Paris while the surgeon carefully molds the foot. The first step is to radically supinate the forefoot to reduce the plantarflexion of the medial column. Once this is achieved, the surgeon applies careful pressure over the talar head while abducting and externally rotating the foot to bring the calcaneus out from under the talus. This process continues with weekly cast changes until the rearfoot is corrected. Then, and only then, can the equinus be addressed. In most cases, management of equinus through manipulation is only partially successful. The residual equinus is corrected by a percutaneous Achilles tenotomy, and casting is continued to maintain the correction (**Fig. 18**). Once these are accomplished, the patient is placed in a brace to maintain correction. This brace may be a simple Fillauer bar and shoe combination or one of several slightly more sophisticated devices that are commercially available. Continued bracing is absolutely necessary for the success of this technique. There are no data to support the fear that the use of bracing following successful reduction of talipes equinovarus by the Ponseti technique adversely influences tibial torsion or femoral antetorsion.[36] Interested readers are referred to Ponseti's monograph on the club foot for details of his clinical management.[37]

Even though the Ponseti technique is highly successful, a few cases still require posteromedial release. There are many variations of this technique, but all include lengthening of the tendo Achilles, posterior ankle and subtalar capsular release, lengthening of tibialis posterior, flexor hallucis longus, and flexor digitorum longus, first- and second-layer plantar muscle release, and capsular release of the talonavicular and calcaneocuboid joints.

Cavus Deformities

Cavus is characterized by high arched deformities, but most are associated with adduction of the forefoot and some degree of inverted heel. The adduction component of the forefoot produces intoeing. The only exception to this is calcaneocavus deformity

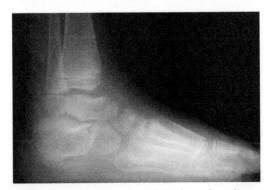

Fig. 17. Residual deformity following posteromedial release for talipes equinovarus. The talar dome is flattened, the talonavicular and calcaneocuboid articulations are malaligned, and forefoot supination remains.

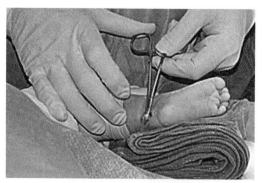

Fig. 18. As the final step in the management of the equinus deformity in talipes equinovarus, the tendo Achilles is sectioned completely under direct vision.

produced by paralysis of the triceps mechanism, resulting in a "pistol-grip" foot deformity. It is doubtful that there are any congenital idiopathic forms of pes cavus or any variation of pes cavus that does not have its origin in some form of neuromuscular disease.

Etiology

Cavus deformities are produced by muscle imbalance, and is the characteristic lesion of Charcot-Marie-Tooth syndrome (**Fig. 19**). Just about any condition that produces muscle imbalance can result in a cavus deformity. These disorders include primary myopathies (Duchenne muscular dystrophy), hereditary peripheral nerve disease (hereditary sensory motor neuropathies), tethered cord, myelomeningocele, syringomyelia, and anterior horn cells disease (**Fig. 20**). Because the underlying etiology may have more serious medical repercussions than the foot and gait problem, obviously this puts a heavy burden on the physician to seek out the cause of this deformity before embarking on any treatment.

Clinical appearance

Stance and gait patterns show internal rotation of the foot to the line of progression as the result of the adducted forefoot that almost always is present with cavus deformities (**Fig. 21**).

The initial step in evaluating the clinical appearance is to determine whether the deformity is flexible or rigid. Simple evaluation of the subtalar range of motion answers

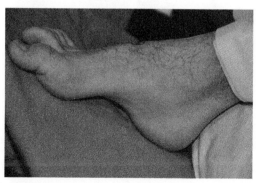

Fig. 19. The typical cavoadductovarus foot appearance in a 19-year-old male patient with Charcot-Marie-Tooth syndrome IA.

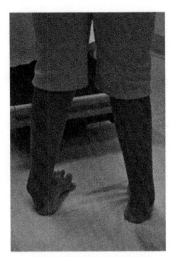

Fig. 20. Bilateral cavovarus deformity in a 5-year-old girl with syringomyelia.

this question. The second step is to evaluate the plantarflexion of the metatarsals. Evaluation for forefoot valgus determines the presence of fixed plantarflexion of all or part of the medial column. Evaluation of the subtalar range of motion and the Coleman Block test identify fixed calcaneal inversion. Clinical examination will give a great deal of information, but radiographs are necessary (**Fig. 22**). Contracture of the plantar fascia can be assessed by palpation. Evaluation of the relationship of the forefoot to rearfoot almost always shows some degree of forefoot valgus. Subtalar range of motion may be near normal or fixed in varus.

Treatment
It is beyond the scope of this article to go into great detail on management, although a few points can be made. Release of the plantar fascia helps reduce the cavus

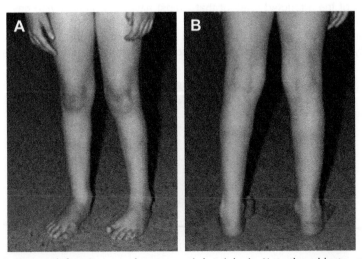

Fig. 21. Cavovarus deformity secondary to spastic hemiplegia. Note the adductus and varus forefoot (*A*) and the fixed inverted heel (*B*).

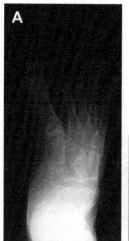
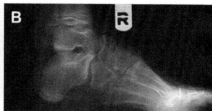

Fig. 22. (A) Anteroposterior projection of right cavus deformity. Note the adduction of the forefoot and the extremely narrow talocalcaneal angle. (B) Lateral projection of right cavus deformity. The talus is maximally dorsiflexed in the ankle. The fibula appears posteriorly displaced because of the adducted forefoot. The first metatarsal is excessively plantarflexed.

deformity. Lateralizing calcaneal osteotomy helps reduce the heel varus. Midfoot osteotomies may be beneficial. The Cole procedure removes a wedge from the dorsal midfoot,[38] but its biggest disadvantage is that it shortens an already short foot. Japas[39] described a V-osteotomy with its apex at the peak of the cavus deformity. Its disadvantage is that it does not allow for any transverse forefoot correction. The Akron dome osteotomy allows for transverse plane correction.[40] Often a dorsiflexing osteotomy of the first metatarsal may be all that is needed to reduce the forefoot valgus. Tibialis posterior is most likely to be the deforming muscle, and transfer through the interosseous ligament to the third cuneiform restores balance.

Summary of Foot and Ankle Disorders

Most of the conditions already discussed are present very early, and should be evident in infants long before they begin to stand and walk. Hallux varus and metatarsus adductus may be completely masked by shoes, and therefore will not produce a significant alteration in gait. The mere appearance of the foot out of shoes is usually enough to make the diagnosis. Management of talipes equinovarus is well documented, but requires considerable training and experience to be successful. Cavus deformities may be present in infants and small children with specific neurologic or neuromuscular etiology. In children with peripheral neuropathy, cavus deformity is more likely to appear toward the end of the first decade of life and is usually a progressive deformity.

Tibial Torsion

Tibial abnormalities are common causes for intoeing gait between the ages of 1 and 2 years. There has been much confusion about both the types and terminology, but the simplest way to understand it is to regard it as an abnormal relationship between the knee axis and the ankle-joint axis. The knee axis is very easy to identify but this is not true for the ankle axis, because there are no external markings defining the axis directly. For this reason, most clinicians use a line passing between the tips of the medial and lateral malleoli (the transmalleolar axis) as a substitute for the true ankle-joint axis. Although the transmalleolar axis does not truly represent the ankle-joint axis itself, it suffices because any error introduced is canceled out by the repetition of the technique. In children older than 2 years, the transmalleolar axis is externally rotated about 15° to 25° to the knee-joint axis. If the remainder of the limb is normal, this should produce an outtoeing gait. Lack of sufficient spontaneous external rotation of the distal tibia will result in some degree of intoeing.

It is important to keep in mind that the angular value is not a constant from birth, but changes rapidly between birth and age 2 years. At birth, tibial torsion is 20° to 30° internal, meaning that the ankle axis is internally rotated about 20° to 30° to the knee axis. Over the first year of life the angle changes (coincidental with the onset of ambulation) so that the ankle axis should be externally rotated about 10° to 12° at 1 year of age. By age 2, tibial torsion should be about 15° to 20° external. By age 5, there is very little additional change as the child reaches most of the adult norm. Abnormal internal tibial torsion does not seem to have any particular gender or side preference.[41]

It is important to remember that some degree of internal tibial torsion is normal in early infancy, and is almost always close to symmetric. When large numbers of children are examined, most will show about 5° more external tibial torsion on the right side than the left. There does not seem to be any explanation for this observation. Most cases of pathologic internal tibial torsion are initially identified between the ages of 1 and 2 years by the development of an intoeing gait.

Etiology
The cause of failure to develop normal external tibial torsion is unknown. It is presumed that most internal tibial torsion is caused by a failure of the lower limb to rotate out at the appropriate rate. Some may be the result of positioning in utero. The problem does tend to run in families, so a genetic component should be considered. There is a relationship between internal tibial torsion and tibia varum so that the two very often go hand in hand. Some degree of tibia varum is physiologic up to age of 2 years. Pathologic tibia varum is related to abnormal development of the proximal tibial metaphysis. This fact puts the burden on the clinician to be certain that there is no intrinsic upper tibial metaphyseal disease. More specific causes include Blount disease and the various forms of rickets.

Clinical appearance
Gait abnormality resulting from internal tibial torsion is very distinctive, and is characterized by internal rotation of the foot to the line of progression while the knee axis is in the coronal plane or slightly externally rotated to it (**Fig. 23**). This definition presumes that there are no other rotational abnormalities in the limb.

There are several ways of estimating tibial torsion. Measurement of the thigh-foot angle is done by placing the child prone on the examining table, flexing the knee at right angles to the table, and evaluating the long axis of the foot against the axis of the thigh (**Fig. 24**). This construct purports to measure tibial torsion, but abnormalities in the foot (adducting, abducting, pronating, or supinating) will adversely affect the measurement. A better method is to place the child supine on the examining table, flex the hip and the knee at right angles, and place the femur vertical in all planes. This positioning puts the knee axis in the plane of the examining table. By very gently externally rotating the tibia on the flexed knee, duplicating the tibiofemoral relationship of the extended knee, the transmalleolar axis is measured against the horizontal with a gravity goniometer or some similar device, thus measuring the transmalleolar axis against the knee axis. Although this does not measure the knee-axis relationship to

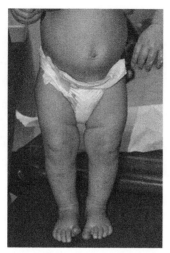

Fig. 23. Internal tibial torsion. Both feet are in the line of progression, but the knees are externally rotated.

the ankle-joint axis directly, the measurement is within 10°, is clinically useful, and is reproducible (**Fig. 25**).

Treatment

The necessity for treating tibial torsion is one of the most controversial topics in the orthopedic literature. The literature maintains that tibial torsion spontaneously reduces. There is no question that the greatest number of cases improves. However, there are many cases of persistent internal tibial torsion with gait abnormalities in older children (**Fig. 26**). Because all cases do not spontaneously correct, the greatest challenge is in identifying those that will not. A few considerations are helpful. First, the younger the infant, the more likely it is that tibial torsion will normalize by age 5 years. Second, the order of magnitude needs to be considered. Large degrees of internal tibial torsion, particularly in older children, are unlikely to correct. Third, symmetry

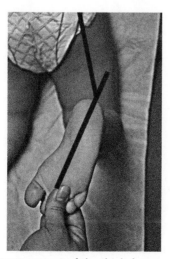

Fig. 24. Positioning for the measurement of the thigh-foot angle.

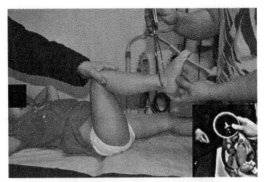

Fig. 25. Measurements of the transmalleolar axis to the knee axis. The patient is placed supine on the examining table. The femur is vertical in all planes. The tibia is gently externally rotated to resistance, and the transmalleolar axis is measured by placing the tips of the gravity goniometer on the medial and lateral malleolar tips (*inset*).

between the two sides needs to be considered. Large abnormalities on one side are unlikely to fully correct. Fourth, internal tibial torsion in children approaching age 2 years is less likely to correct. Fifth, an important consideration is that the success of nonoperative management of tibial torsion decreases as the child approaches age 2. Consequently, persisting internal tibial torsion past that age will either have to be accepted or corrected by tibial osteotomy, if indicated. Sixth, internal tibial torsion associated with talipes equinovarus rarely improves spontaneously, and tends to be unresponsive to nonoperative treatment (**Fig. 27**).

It is appropriate to take a watch-and-wait approach in children younger than 1 year. The probability of natural correction is high, and there still is a wide window of opportunity for successful nonoperative treatment if there is no evidence of improvement. Between the ages of 12 and 15 months, infants with tibial torsion very often respond to the use of transverse bars at night and naptime. The bars do not force the extremities into external rotation in an attempt to "torque" the tibia out, but rather function to

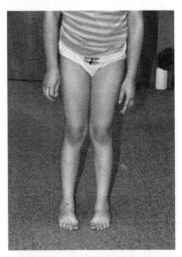

Fig. 26. Persistent internal tibial torsion in a 7-year-old girl. Note the internal rotation of the feet while the patellae are directed straight ahead.

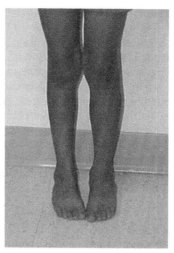

Fig. 27. Persistent internal tibial torsion in a child with successful treatment of talipes equinovarus. Note the small right calf and the dimple over the sinus tarsi.

prevent the assumption of internal rotating positions during sleep that perpetuate the deformity. Past the age of 15 months, a more aggressive approach should be instituted. Serial casting is the gold standard with which all other therapies is compared. A long leg cast is applied with the knee flexed about 45°. The cast is applied from the groin to an area approximately 3 cm above the ankle. After this component of the cast hardens, a foot and ankle component is applied with the rearfoot in neutral position, the ankle plantarflexed, and a gap left between the two portions of the cast. Once this has hardened, the two segments of the cast are joined together with the foot externally rotated in the cast. This technique is reminiscent of the transverse plane control used by the Ponseti method for clubfoot management. After a week, the cast is circularized just above the ankle and the foot component is externally rotated further. The cast is repaired. After an additional week, the entire cast is removed and replaced as described earlier. This sequence continues until tibial torsion has normalized for the age. Follow-up with a transverse bar at night and naptime for about 4 months after successful cast reduction minimizes the likelihood of recurrence.

Persisting tibial torsion past the age of 2 years is unlikely to respond to nonoperative therapy, and is also less likely to spontaneously correct. In the presence of significant gait disturbance, the options are to accept the deformity if possible or correct it with tibial osteotomy. Tibial osteotomy can be performed at either the upper tibia or lower tibia. Operations on the lower tibia are considered safer than proximal tibial osteotomies because of the fear of compartment syndrome, damage to the common peroneal nerve and the major neurovascular structures posterior to the upper tibia. These surgical concerns favor supramalleolar osteotomy.[42,43] A dome-shaped osteotomy done either proximally or distally, depending on the severity of the deformity, may be indicated when there is internal tibial torsion associated with varus deformity of the tibia.[44]

THE PELVIS AND THE PROXIMAL FEMUR
The Acetabulum

The physical examination of neonates and infants generates a contradiction between what is known about the anatomy of the femur and what is found on the examination of range of motion of the hip. When the infant's hips are in extension, internal rotation of the extremities is about 20° and external rotation 40° to 50°. At the same time, it is known that the relationship of the proximal femur to the distal femur (femoral anteversion, femoral antetorsion, medial femoral torsion; see later discussion) is such that intoeing should be the limb position. Instead, the infant assumes a flexed, abducted, and externally rotated posture (**Fig. 28**). It has been postulated that the explanation for this lies in physiologic contracture secondary to in utero position, and that with time this contracture disappears. As the infant becomes older, the direction of rotation changes. The total range of motion remains about 60° to 70°, but with time internal rotation becomes greater at the expense of loss of external rotation. If the hypothesis regarding periacetabular ligament contracture is correct, it is expected that internal rotation would increase. However, the weakness of this theory is that external rotation decreases with time as the amount of internal rotation increases, thus suggesting that another factor is operating.

Acetabular anteversion and retroversion

It has been suggested that the acetabulum changes position on the pelvis over time. It would be attractive to assume that the acetabulum is directed more posteriolaterally (retroverted) in the infant, and over time rotates into a more anterolateral position (becoming anteverted). The literature is highly divided on this. Part of the problem with proving or disproving this concept is that imaging of the acetabulum to determine its relative position is very difficult. Even with the use of magnetic resonance imaging and computed tomography, it is difficult to prove or disprove this theory. There is some support for the concept of acetabular anteversion and retroversion from the literature dealing with reconstruction of hip dysplasia by pelvic osteotomy.[45] The term combined anteversion was coined to indicate acetabular anteversion plus femoral anteversion (antetorsion).[46] Certain combined visceral and pelvic anomalies such as bladder exstrophy are known to have altered orientation of the acetabulum.[47]

The position of the head of the femur in the acetabulum

The head of the femur rotates more or less freely in the acetabulum in the transverse body plane. If the head-neck–greater trochanter (HNGT) axis is considered the

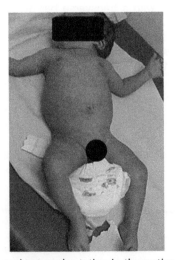

Fig. 28. Flexion, abduction, and external rotation in the resting infant.

reference, there are an infinite number of positions of the HNGT axis related to the coronal or frontal plane of the body throughout the range of hip motion. If the HNGT axis is in the frontal or coronal plane, the proximal femur is neither anteverted nor retroverted in the acetabulum. If the femur is externally rotated in the acetabulum, the HNGT axis runs in an anteromedial direction and is anteverted, resulting in external rotation of the entire limb. If the femur is internally rotated, the proximal femur is retroverted and the entire limb is internally rotated. The only time that this would take on clinical significance would be if the soft tissues around the acetabulum (muscle and ligament) actually do become contracted. Under these circumstances, the proximal femur would be held in an abnormal position.

Returning to the ranges of motion in the infant, during the neonatal examination the lower extremities assume a passive abduction, flexion, and external rotation position. The proximal femur then is anteverted in the acetabulum, even though the limb is now in external rotation (see **Fig. 28**).

The relationship of the femoral head to the neck

The relationship of the functional articular surface of the head of the femur on its neck is another poorly explored concept. The presumption that it is placed on the neck at right angles may or may not be correct. It is possible that the usable articular surface could be rotated anteriorly (anteverted) or posteriorly (retroverted). As an example, in patients with slipped capital femoral epiphysis, the head is no longer in an appropriate position on the neck, which results in the figure-4 phenomenon on clinical examination (external rotation of the femur when the hip is flexed in the sagittal plane). The entire limb is externally rotated (**Fig. 29**). The possibility of acetabular retroversion developing in children with slipped capital femoral epiphysis as they enter adulthood has been documented.[48]

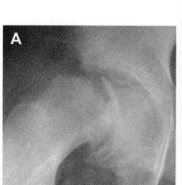
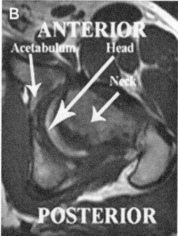

Fig. 29. Slipped capital femoral epiphysis. (*A*) Plain radiograph shows the displacement of the femoral head. (*B*) Magnetic resonance image of the same patient shows the femoral head in the acetabulum, but the neck and greater trochanter are rotated anteriorly, placing the limb in external rotation; this results in a functional fixed anteversion. (*Courtesy of* Laurie Lomasney, MD, Department of Radiology, Loyola University Medical Center, Maywood, IL.)

Femoral Anteversion (Antetorsion, Medial Femoral Torsion)

In the general orthopedic literature, femoral antetorsion, femoral anteversion, and medial femoral torsion are used interchangeably. However, the whole issue of rotational abnormalities originating in the proximal femur, its relationship to the acetabulum, and acetabular position on the pelvis is much more complex. Anteversion and retroversion are applied to several different and unrelated concepts, leading to confusion about the meaning of these 2 terms.

There is precedent already set for making a distinction between the terms femoral anteversion and femoral antetorsion. Common usage in the podiatry and physical therapy literature defines femoral anteversion as the angle formed by the HNGT axis and the frontal or coronal plane of the body, whereas antetorsion refers to the angle formed by the HNGT axis and the transcondylar axis of the distal femur. Stated another way, femoral antetorsion measures the osseous "twist" between the upper femur and lower femur, whereas anteversion describes the momentary position of the femur in the acetabulum or defines the relative position of the acetabulum on the pelvis. The same is true for retrotorsion and retroversion.

The HNGT axis is not parallel to the axis of the knee joint (determined by measuring the transcondylar axis). Data suggest that the HNGT axis is always transversely rotated anteromedial to the transcondylar line. In early fetal development, it is a very small angle (about 5°–7°). It is largest in term infants, at 30° to 38°. It then falls gradually throughout childhood and adolescence, finally reaching the adult value of approximately 15° to 20°.[49] Its highest values are between birth and 30 months of age. This anteromedial direction of the HNGT axis is variously referred to as femoral anteversion, femoral antetorsion, and medial femoral torsion. However, because the term anteversion can also designate the position of the acetabulum on the pelvis as well as momentary position of the proximal femur within the acetabulum, it seems less confusing to follow the physical therapy literature and use the terms antetorsion and retrotorsion to describe the relationship between the HNGT axis of the femur and the distal femur, and use the term anteversion and retroversion to describe everything else. The data described here regarding the angular values also strongly suggest that the reversal of the HNGT axis to the transcondylar axis so that the proximal portion runs in a posteromedial direction is never physiologic and is very unusual.[50] There are no studies that establish that femoral retrotorsion is a part of the normal development of the lower limb at or after birth. Therefore, retrotorsion should be considered pathologic at any age.

There is a relationship between increased angles of femoral antetorsion and coxa valga (defined as the angle formed by the shaft of the femur and the head and neck axis in the coronal plane). When viewed on the coronal plane, the angle formed by the long axis of the shaft with the head-neck axis starts out at about 150° in infancy, and then slowly decreases over the first 2 decades until reaching the normal adult value of about 120°. This angle is known as the angle of inclination. Values above and below the norm for the age are called coxa valgum and coxa varum, respectively.

Etiology

The cause of pathologic femoral antetorsion is unknown, but the natural history of spontaneous correction is well documented.[51] Most cases of femoral antetorsion have normalized by age 8 years.[52] The explanation for persistence is open to speculation. The child's neurologic status is the first issue to be considered. Neurologically normal children are highly likely to spontaneously correct. Neurologically abnormal children from whatever cause have a much lower incidence of spontaneous correction, and often actually worsen with time. Abnormal femoral antetorsion frequently runs in families, raising the possibility of an inherited trait. The gender ratio is skewed toward females.[41,53] The "television-sitting" or W-sitting position is also implicated.[54] This W-sitting position keeps the hips internally rotated. Sitting with the feet under the buttocks not only internally rotates the femurs but also both internally rotates the tibias and adducts the forefoot (**Fig. 30**).

Neurologic abnormality is a quite different situation. The child with cerebral palsy is the best model for this type of intoeing. Internal rotation and scissoring are common gait changes in children with spasticity and hypertonia.[55] Factors thought to contribute to the abnormal gait include femoral antetorsion, hip-flexor tightness, imbalance of hip rotators and other muscles,[56] and hamstring and adductor tightness. Fixed anatomic abnormalities occur, and are not amenable to any therapy other than surgical derotation osteotomy. Dynamic internal rotation of the hip, on the other hand, is multifactorial in origin.[57] Unlike the neurologically normal children whose angles of

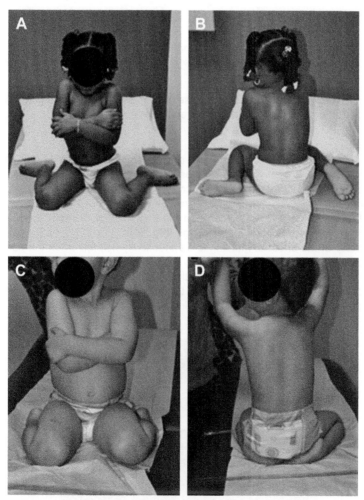

Fig. 30. (*A, B*) The W-sitting or television-sitting position with the legs externally rotated. (*C, D*) A similar position with the feet tucked under the buttocks accentuating the internal tibial torsion as well as metatarsus adductus.

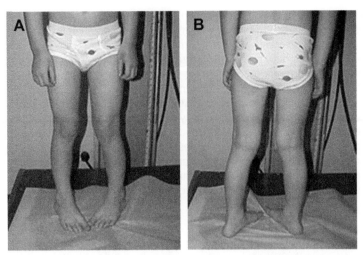

Fig. 31. Femoral antetorsion. Note the internal rotation of the patellae (squinting patella sign) (*A*), and internal rotation of the popliteal creases when viewed from the posterior (*B*).

femoral antetorsion progressively decrease, the angle shows little change and may actually become greater in children with cerebral palsy.[58]

Clinical appearance

Given the presumption that the remainder of the lower extremity is normal, abnormal amounts of femoral antetorsion cause intoeing. This appearance is easily recognized in gait observation because the popliteal creases and, to a lesser extent, the patellae are rotated internally. This rotation is consistent throughout the stance-and-swing phase of gait. In bipedal stance, because the entire femur is internally rotated, the patellae assume the "squinting patella" sign (**Fig. 31**).

The history of the onset of intoeing is diagnostically helpful. Often the parents will relate that the child's gait has been more or less normal up until roughly about the age of 2 years. At that time, the family notices sudden development of intoeing. The reason for this is speculated to be related to the change of the direction of the range of hip motion between the time the child first begins to walk at 1 year and 2 years of

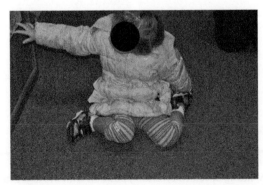

Fig. 32. A 29-month-old female observed in the W-sitting position while in the reception area before the examination.

age. It must be borne in mind that hip rotation in extension is changing from relative external rotation to internal rotation, which thus unmasks the abnormal femoral ante-torsion that has always been present.

The child favors the W-sitting position. This position can be observed while the child is playing in the reception room, and suggests the diagnosis even before the physician begins the examination (**Fig. 32**).

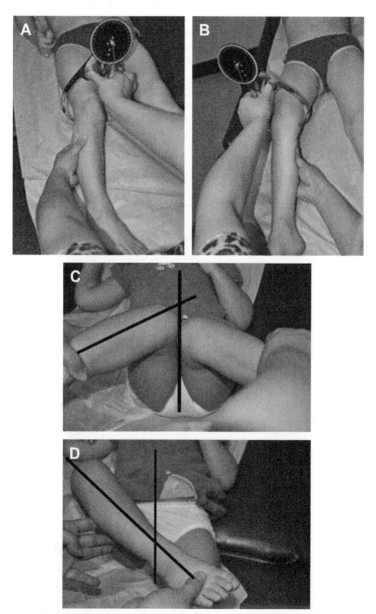

Fig. 33. Measurement of internal (A) and external (B) rotation of the hip in extension. (C) Measurement of internal rotation of the hip in the flexed position. (D) Measurement of external rotation of the hip in the hip-flexed position.

Examining range of motion of the hip in extension and flexion helps confirm the diagnosis of femoral antetorsion. Regularly there will be a great deal of internal rotation of the hips in comparison with external rotation when measured in the hip-extended position. There may be as much as 60° of internal rotation and as little as 10° to 15° of external rotation. Rotation must also be evaluated with the thighs flexed at right angles on the trunk. Internal rotation often remains unchanged while external rotation increases. Generally speaking, external rotation in flexion less than 45° is confirmatory. Higher values of antetorsion will further limit external rotation in flexion (**Fig. 33**).[59] On occasion, a child with limited external rotation in extension may demonstrate near normal external hip rotation in the hip-flexed position, but this does not alter the diagnosis. Rotation can also be measured with the child in the prone position, the hips extended, and the knees flexed (**Fig. 34**).

There are several methods for determining the angle of femoral antetorsion without having to resort to computer-assisted imaging. The first method is simple and is known as the Ryder maneuver.[60] The child is placed in the supine position. The greater trochanter is palpated through the skin, and the thigh is internally and externally rotated several times until the examiner feels that the HNGT axis has been leveled and is in the plane of the examining table. A gravity goniometer or similar device is used to measure the position of the transcondylar axis of the knee. If the transcondylar axis of the knee is rotated internally, this is an antetorsion value. If, for some reason (a pathologic one), the distal femur is externally rotated, this is a retrotorsion value (**Fig. 35**).

A second technique can be used if no instrumentation is available. The child is placed prone on the examining table and, in the same manner described above, the greater trochanter is palpated until the proximal anatomy is level with the examination table. The angle that the tibia forms with the vertical is then measured. If the tibia is externally rotated, this corresponds to an antetorsion value; if it is internally rotated, it corresponds to a retrotorsion value. The angle measured is called the trochanteric prominence angle (**Fig. 36**).[61–63] This technique has been studied in children with cerebral palsy, and several conclusions have been reached. First, the test correlates well with radiographic determination and can be used for routine clinical determination.

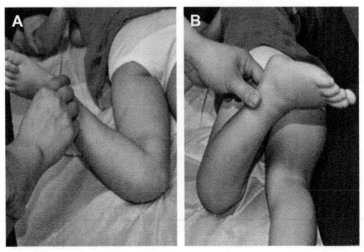

Fig. 34. Measurement of internal (*A*) and external (*B*) rotation of the hip in the prone position with the hip extended and the knee flexed.

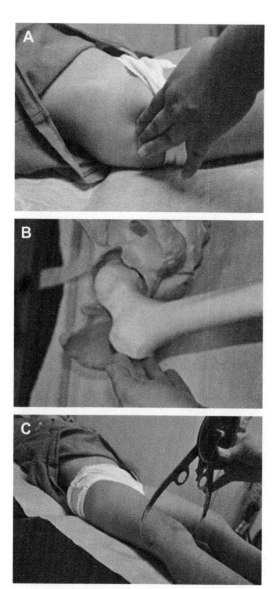

Fig. 35. Ryder maneuver. The greater trochanter is palpated through the skin, and the thigh is rotated internally and externally until the examiner feels that he has leveled the head-neck–greater trochanter axis (*A*); this is demonstrated on a skeletal specimen (*B*). (*C*) Ryder maneuver, continued. The transmalleolar axis is measured with a gravity goniometer. Because the distal femur was internally rotated, this is an antetorsion value.

Second, hip rotation in flexion had a better correlation with radiographic antetorsion measurement, and clinical examination in hips flexed 90° allows for better assessment of femoral anteversion than examination done in hip extension.[62]

Treatment
Of course, nonoperative management of intoeing problems caused by femoral ante-torsion would be highly advantageous. There would be virtually no risk. The cost factor

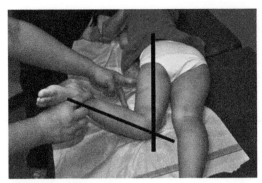

Fig. 36. The trochanteric prominence angle. The child is placed prone and the thigh is rotated in and out as in the Ryder maneuver, until the head-neck–greater trochanter axis is leveled. The angle formed by the leg and the vertical is then measured as the angle of antetorsion.

would be negligible in comparison with surgical intervention. There would be no particular skill required on the part of the physician. Nonoperative treatments proposed include braces, wedges, stretches and exercises, shoe modifications, and other orthotic devices. Unfortunately there is little supportive evidence that any of these methods are of any benefit,[64–66] which holds especially true for shoes, shoe modifications, and in-shoe orthoses.[67,68]

Physical therapy techniques are based on the erroneous concept that the persistent internal rotation of the limb is due to tight capsular ligaments. Nighttime bars and bracing have not proved to be effective. Twister cables may modify gait while worn, but do not correct or even modify the natural history of antetorsion. Adaptations of shoes and devices worn inside the shoes to promote outtoeing are cosmetic at best, do not modify the natural history of the condition, and often fail to improve the gait. In some cases, intoeing actually worsens with these devices. Orthoses that are designed to reverse intoeing have one other disadvantage. For external rotation of the foot to occur when the more proximal limb is fixed in internal rotation, the subtalar and midtarsal joints have to pronate in the later portions of the stance phase of gait; this is contrary to the desired response of supinating during heel-off. Routine use of orthoses for fixed internal gait disturbances caused by femoral antetorsion and internal tibial torsion should be abandoned as ineffective and nonphysiologic.

Surgical management of femoral antetorsion is an option for selected cases, based on severity and neurologic status. Derotation osteotomy in the proximal or distal femur allows reduction of the angle of femoral antetorsion. However, this is a somewhat involved procedure and carries the potential for significant complications[11] including undercorrection and overcorrection, malunion and nonunion of the femur, potential for infection, compartment syndrome, and issues with retained hardware. Moreover, postoperative convalescence is time consuming. In neurologically normal children, this type of therapy is indicated only in children who have severe negative impact on activities of daily living.[52] In addition, consideration for surgical intervention should be delayed until age 10 to 12 years, when the potential for spontaneous improvement has run its course.[1,11]

The decision to intervene in children with cerebral palsy is more straightforward. Unlike neurologically normal children, they do not follow the natural history of spontaneous correction and have the potential for worsening. Femoral derotation osteotomy is the preferred treatment.[69] The association of femoral antetorsion and coxa valga is very high, and this combination puts the hip at risk for subluxation and dislocation. Derotation osteotomy can be combined with varus osteotomy. The movement disorders characteristic of cerebral palsy also complicate the development and maturation of gait and lead to dysfunction.[70] Derotation can be performed either in the proximal femur above or below the lesser trochanter[69] or in the distal femur.

Miserable malalignment syndrome, sometimes referred to as malignant malalignment syndrome, is a combination of severe femoral antetorsion and marked pathologic external tibial torsion. Although the combination of the two often balances gait so that there is little or no abnormal foot-progression angle, the net effect is patellofemoral dysfunction, and many of these children have patellar pain in the form of chondromalacia patellae, sometimes ending in subluxation. Many of these patients are resistant to nonoperative treatment.[71–73]

SUMMARY

Diagnosis and treatment of intoeing may seem problematic, but is really quite simple because there are only a handful of pathologic conditions that need to be considered. The workup is also made simple because the causes of intoeing are limited to 3 anatomic areas. Issues within the foot are easily identified, and are amenable to surgical and nonsurgical treatment. The other 2 areas are the tibiofibular segment and the femur itself. These last 2 areas are therapeutically difficult, and are also complicated by the fact that there is a well-defined natural history for spontaneous correction that must be taken into consideration, recognizing that the natural history does not guarantee a successful outcome. There are some nonsurgical interventions that may be used for tibial torsion, but there are no nonoperative treatments for femoral antetorsion. Issues with the position of the acetabulum on the pelvis are as yet unstudied, and no conclusions can be drawn about their clinical significance.

Management of intoeing is subject to the same rules of evidence-based medicine as for any other medical treatment. It is necessary to select therapies based on the likelihood of success. Regarding problems in the feet, the success of nonoperative management of conditions such as metatarsus adductus and talipes equinovarus is well documented. For such nonresponsive cases, surgical salvage is also well recognized.

Management of tibial torsion is extremely controversial. Nonoperative techniques such as bar therapy and serial casting are used, with some success. The real issue is the identification of cases that will not spontaneously correct, because clinical experience clearly shows that not all cases do. Those children who have not followed the rule of spontaneous correction are locked in a difficult situation. The amount of intoeing usually is enough to be objectionable, but not enough to justify the risk of derotation osteotomy. Selection criteria must be developed so that children who are at risk for failure of spontaneous resolution can be identified and treated at an appropriate age, if possible, to ensure success.

Persistent femoral antetorsion is an even greater dilemma because there are no nonoperative treatments available. Avoidance of the W-sitting position is logical, but its effect on the natural history is unknown. The real issue here is determining which children need surgery. The neurologically abnormal children are much easier to deal with because the persistence of femoral antetorsion not only results in a disturbance of walking but also places the hip at risk for dislocation.

Although there would be great interest in managing tibial torsion and femoral antetorsion nonoperatively, it must be kept in mind that there really are no universally successful techniques; this raises the issue of conservative versus radical treatment. If it is accepted that that there are no nonoperative therapies, the use of bracing and other techniques becomes radical and unscientific, given that there is no potential for success. Surgical management then becomes conservative.

As a final note, most intoeing in toddlers and older children is not caused by abnormality within the foot. Tibial torsion and femoral antetorsion are the 2 most common diagnoses. Beyond the age of 2 years, femoral antetorsion dominates. However, within the last 3 or 4 years, this author has noticed an increase in the incidence in children aged 5 to 12 years. From the therapeutic perspective, it must be realized that there are no in-shoe devices that will correct or modify the natural history of these 2 disorders. This aspect is especially important because parents intuitively seek out foot and ankle specialists when their children intoe. The burden is then placed on the examiner to recognize the causes of intoeing and to prescribe therapy accordingly.

REFERENCES

1. Terjesen T, Svenningsen S. Idiopathic femur anteversion. Tidsskr Nor Laegeforen 1995;115:2381 [in Norwegian].
2. Blackmur JP, Murray AW. Do children who in-toe need to be referred to an orthopaedic clinic? J Pediatr Orthop B 2010;19:415.
3. Li YH, Leong JC. Intoeing gait in children. Hong Kong Med J 1999;5:360.
4. Aston JW Jr. In-toeing gait in children. Am Fam Physician 1979;19:111.
5. Furdon SA, Donlon CR. Examination of the newborn foot: positional and structural abnormalities. Adv Neonatal Care 2002;2:248.
6. Katz K, David R, Soudry M. Below-knee plaster cast for the treatment of metatarsus adductus. J Pediatr Orthop 1999;19:49.
7. Bielski RJ, Gesell MW, Teng AL, et al. Orthopaedic implications of multiple gestation pregnancy with triplets. J Pediatr Orthop 2006;26:129.
8. Hensinger RN. Rotational problems of the lower extremity. Postgrad Med 1976; 60:161.
9. Bleck EE. Developmental orthopaedics. III: Toddlers. Dev Med Child Neurol 1982;24:533.
10. Charvat J. Metatarsus varus among forefoot adduction deformities in children. Acta Chir Orthop Traumatol Cech 1996;63:221 [in Czech].
11. Dietz FR. Intoeing—fact, fiction and opinion. Am Fam Physician 1994;50:1249.
12. Karol LA. Rotational deformities in the lower extremities. Curr Opin Pediatr 1997; 9:77.
13. Killam PE. Orthopedic assessment of young children: developmental variations. Nurse Pract 1989;14:27.
14. Sass P, Hassan G. Lower extremity abnormalities in children. Am Fam Physician 2003;68:461.
15. Lincoln TL, Suen PW. Common rotational variations in children. J Am Acad Orthop Surg 2003;11:312.
16. Kim HD, Lee DS, Eom MJ, et al. Relationship between physical examinations and two-dimensional computed tomographic findings in children with intoeing gait. Ann Rehabil Med 2011;35:491.
17. Staheli LT. In-toeing and out-toeing in children. J Fam Pract 1983;16:1005.
18. Staheli LT, Corbett M, Wyss C, et al. Lower-extremity rotational problems in children. Normal values to guide management. J Bone Joint Surg Am 1985;67:39.
19. Lichtblau S. Section of the abductor hallucis tendon for correction of metatarsus varus deformity. Clin Orthop Relat Res 1975;227.
20. Mubarak SJ, O'Brien TJ, Davids JR. Metatarsal epiphyseal bracket: treatment by central physiolysis. J Pediatr Orthop 1993;13:5.

21. Shea KG, Mubarak SJ, Alamin T. Preossified longitudinal epiphyseal bracket of the foot: treatment by partial bracket excision before ossification. J Pediatr Orthop 2001;21:360.

22. Heyman CH, Herndon CH, Strong JM. Mobilization of the tarsometatarsal and intertarsal joints for the correction of resistant adduction of the fore part of the foot in congenital club-foot or congenital metatarsus varus. J Bone Joint Surg Am 1958;40:299.

23. Jawish R, Rigault P, Padovani JP, et al. The Z-shaped or serpentine foot in children and adolescents. Chir Pediatr 1990;31:314 [in French].

24. Peterson HA. Skewfoot (forefoot adduction with heel valgus). J Pediatr Orthop 1986;6:24.

25. Wan SC. Metatarsus adductus and skewfoot deformity. Clin Podiatr Med Surg 2006;23:23.

26. Thompson GH, Simons GW. Congenital talippes equinovarus (clubfeet) and metatarsus adductus. In: Drennan JC, editor. The child's foot and ankle. New York: Raven Press; 1992. p. 97.

27. Ponseti IV, Zhivkov M, Davis N, et al. Treatment of the complex idiopathic clubfoot. Clin Orthop Relat Res 2006;451:171.

28. Howlett JP, Mosca VS, Bjornson K. The association between idiopathic clubfoot and increased internal hip rotation. Clin Orthop Relat Res 2009;467:1231.

29. Herceg MB, Weiner DS, Agamanolis DP, et al. Histologic and histochemical analysis of muscle specimens in idiopathic talipes equinovarus. J Pediatr Orthop 2006;26:91.

30. Isaacs H, Handelsman JE, Badenhorst M, et al. The muscles in club foot—a histological histochemical and electron microscopic study. J Bone Joint Surg Br 1977;59:465.

31. Loren GJ, Karpinski NC, Mubarak SJ. Clinical implications of clubfoot histopathology. J Pediatr Orthop 1998;18:765.

32. Nadeem RD, Brown JK, Lawson G, et al. Somatosensory evoked potentials as a means of assessing neurological abnormality in congenital talipes equinovarus. Dev Med Child Neurol 2000;42:525.

33. Song KS, Kang CH, Min BW, et al. Congenital clubfoot with concomitant peroneal nerve palsy in children. J Pediatr Orthop B 2008;17:85.

34. Thometz J, Sathoff L, Liu XC, et al. Electromyography nerve conduction velocity evaluation of children with clubfeet. Am J Orthop 2011;40:84.

35. Feldbrin Z, Gilai AN, Ezra E, et al. Muscle imbalance in the aetiology of idiopathic club foot. An electromyographic study. J Bone Joint Surg Br 1995;77:596.

36. Boehm S, Sinclair M. Foot abduction brace in the Ponseti method for idiopathic clubfoot deformity: torsional deformities and compliance. J Pediatr Orthop 2007;27:712.

37. Ponseti IV. Congenital clubfoot fundamentals of treatment. Oxford (United Kingdom): Oxford University Press; 1996.

38. Cole WH. The treatment of claw foot. J Bone Joint Surg 1940;22:895.

39. Japas LM. Surgical treatment of pes cavus by tarsal v-osteotomy. J Bone Joint Surg Am 1968;50:927.

40. Wilcox P, Weiner D. Akron midtarsal dome osteotomy in the treatment of rigid pes cavus: a preliminary review. J Pediatr Orthop 1985;5:330.

41. Jacquemier M, Glard Y, Pomero V, et al. Rotational profile of the lower limb in 1319 healthy children. Gait Posture 2008;28:187.

42. Savva N, Ramesh R, Richards RH. Supramalleolar osteotomy for unilateral tibial torsion. J Pediatr Orthop B 2006;15:190.

43. Selber P, Filho ER, Dallalana R, et al. Supramalleolar derotation osteotomy of the tibia, with T plate fixation. Technique and results in patients with neuromuscular disease. J Bone Joint Surg Br 2004;86:1170.

44. Dilawaiz Nadeem R, Quick TJ, Eastwood DM. Focal dome osteotomy for the correction of tibial deformity in children. J Pediatr Orthop B 2005;14:340.

45. Fujii M, Nakashima Y, Sato T, et al. Acetabular tilt correlates with acetabular version and coverage in hip dysplasia. Clin Orthop Relat Res 2012;470:2827.

46. Maheshwari AV, Zlowodzki MP, Siram G, et al. Femoral neck anteversion, acetabular anteversion and combined anteversion in the normal Indian adult population: a computed tomographic study. Indian J Orthop 2010;44:277.

47. Suson KD, Sponseller PD, Gearhart JP. Bony abnormalities in classic bladder exstrophy: the urologist's perspective. J Pediatr Urol 2013;9:112–22.

48. Sankar WN, Flynn JM. The development of acetabular retroversion in children with Legg-Calve-Perthes disease. J Pediatr Orthop 2008;28:440.

49. Shefelbine SJ, Carter DR. Mechanobiological predictions of femoral anteversion in cerebral palsy. Ann Biomed Eng 2004;32:297.

50. Wagner R, Barcak EA. Simultaneous proximal femoral rotational and distal femoral varus osteotomies for femoral retroversion and genu valgum. Am J Orthop (Belle Mead NJ) 2012;41:175.

51. Svenningsen S, Apalset K, Terjesen T, et al. Regression of femoral anteversion. A prospective study of intoeing children. Acta Orthop Scand 1989;60:170.

52. Gordon JE, Pappademos PC, Schoenecker PL, et al. Diaphyseal derotational osteotomy with intramedullary fixation for correction of excessive femoral anteversion in children. J Pediatr Orthop 2005;25:548.

53. Medina McKeon JM, Hertel J. Sex differences and representative values for 6 lower extremity alignment measures. J Athl Train 2009;44:249.

54. Altinel L, Kose KC, Aksoy Y, et al. Hip rotation degrees, intoeing problem, and sitting habits in nursery school children: an analysis of 1,134 cases. Acta Orthop Traumatol Turc 2007;41:190 [in Turkish].

55. Brunner R, Krauspe R, Romkes J. Torsion deformities in the lower extremities in patients with infantile cerebral palsy: pathogenesis and therapy. Orthopade 2000;29:808 [in German].

56. Aktas S, Aiona MD, Orendurff M. Evaluation of rotational gait abnormality in the patients cerebral palsy. J Pediatr Orthop 2000;20:217.

57. O'Sullivan R, Walsh M, Hewart P, et al. Factors associated with internal hip rotation gait in patients with cerebral palsy. J Pediatr Orthop 2006;26:537.

58. Bobroff ED, Chambers HG, Sartoris DJ, et al. Femoral anteversion and neck-shaft angle in children with cerebral palsy. Clin Orthop Relat Res 1999;194.

59. Gelberman RH, Cohen MS, Desai SS, et al. Femoral anteversion. A clinical assessment of idiopathic intoeing gait in children. J Bone Joint Surg Br 1987;69:75.

60. Ryder CT, Crane L. Measuring femoral anteversion; the problem and a method. J Bone Joint Surg Am 1953;35:321.

61. Chung CY, Lee KM, Park MS, et al. Validity and reliability of measuring femoral anteversion and neck-shaft angle in patients with cerebral palsy. J Bone Joint Surg Am 2010;92:1195.

62. Adamczyk E, Sibinski M, Synder M. The value of femoral anteversion angle measured clinically and on radiographs. Chir Narzadow Ruchu Ortop Pol 2010;75:344 [in Polish].

63. Davids JR, Benfanti P, Blackhurst DW, et al. Assessment of femoral anteversion in children with cerebral palsy: accuracy of the trochanteric prominence angle test. J Pediatr Orthop 2002;22:173.

64. Briggs RG, Carlson WO. The management of intoeing: a review. S D J Med 1990;43:13.
65. Redmond AC. An evaluation of the use of gait plate inlays in the short-term management of the intoeing child. Foot Ankle Int 1998;19:144.
66. Uden H, Kumar S. Non-surgical management of a pediatric "intoed" gait pattern—a systematic review of the current best evidence. J Multidiscip Healthc 2012;5:27.
67. Knittel G, Staheli LT. The effectiveness of shoe modifications for intoeing. Orthop Clin North Am 1976;7:1019.
68. Staheli LT, Giffin L. Corrective shoes for children: a survey of current practice. Pediatrics 1980;65:13.
69. de Morais Filho MC, Kawamura CM, dos Santos CA, et al. Outcomes of correction of internal hip rotation in patients with spastic cerebral palsy using proximal femoral osteotomy. Gait Posture 2012;36:201.
70. Turker M, Cirpar M, Cetik O, et al. Comparison of two techniques in achieving planned correction angles in femoral subtrochanteric derotation osteotomy. J Pediatr Orthop B 2012;21:215.
71. Bruce WD, Stevens PM. Surgical correction of miserable malalignment syndrome. J Pediatr Orthop 2004;24:392.
72. Delgado ED, Schoenecker PL, Rich MM, et al. Treatment of severe torsional malalignment syndrome. J Pediatr Orthop 1996;16:484.
73. Garcia-Mata S, Hidalgo-Ovejero A. Primary recurrent medial subdislocation of both patellae. Long-term review of an exceptional case of miserably malalignment syndrome. An Sist Sanit Navar 2007;30:459 [in Spanish].

Congenital Talotarsal Joint Displacement and Pes Planovalgus

Evaluation, Conservative Management, and Surgical Management

Michael E. Graham, DPM, FACFAS, FAENS

KEYWORDS

- Pes planovalgus • Pediatric flatfoot • Subtalar instability
- Congenital talotarsal dislocation • Extraosseous talotarsal stabilization • Orthosis
- Subtalar arthroereisis

KEY POINTS

- Congenital talotarsal displacement is typically a component of pes planovalgus yet this deformity can present without a flat foot.
- Radiographic characteristics of talotarsal displacement show obliteration of the sinus tarsi as the primary finding. Additional findings include sagittal and/or transverse plane components.
- Early treatment intervention is preferred, as this dynamic deformity has been named as the primary underlying cause of many foot and ankle deformities.
- Conservative care is very limited in its ability to stabilize the talotarsal joint and thus prevent the progression of the disease process.
- When indicated, minimal invasive treatment options, such as extraosseous talotarsal stabilization, are preferred to reconstructive surgical options for flexible deformities.

INTRODUCTION

A range of treatment protocols for pediatric flatfoot have been presented in the scientific literature. There seems to be no common consensus on the best treatment modality, and, if history teaches us anything, it is unlikely there ever will be an accepted consensus. However, there is agreement on the importance of a stable hindfoot to the biomechanics of the foot and ankle, as well as to the proximal musculoskeletal chain. Although some investigators argue that ligament or other soft-tissue laxity plays

Disclosures: M.E. Graham is the inventor of HyProCure, the President & Founder of the Graham International Implant Institute and the sole owner of GraMedica, LLC, which manufactures and distributes HyProCure nationally and internationally. He lectures on an ongoing basis about HyProCure to foot surgeons worldwide.
Graham International Implant Institute, 16137 Leone Drive, Macomb, MI 48042, USA
E-mail address: mgraham@gramedica.com

a significant role in hindfoot instability, it is commonly accepted that soft-tissue connections play a secondary role at best, and are more likely a sequela resulting from an osseous malformation. Flexible flatfoot is essentially the result of the partial dislocation(s) of 1 or more joints within the talotarsal mechanism. The talotarsal mechanism is composed of the talus, the navicular, the calcaneus, and the 4 joints formed by the articulations of these bones (talonavicular and middle, anterior, and posterior talocalcaneal, or subtalar joint). It has been stated that "symptoms can be relieved, and the functions of the foot restored only by a reduction of the misplaced bones and their retention in normal position."[1] Too often, treatment is aimed only at the amelioration of any presenting symptoms while the underlying etiology is ignored or untreated. While there is much discussion about preventive medicine, in actuality very little attention is directed toward that goal. In particular, the majority of the Pediatrics medical community has ignored, or paid very little attention to, the alignment of the foot.[2] Many assume that a misaligned hindfoot is an acceptable deformity that will most likely resolve on its own.[3] The reality is that the deformity will continually progress, eventually leading to secondary deformities not only in the foot and ankle, but up the musculoskeletal chain.

PARTIAL TALOTARSAL DISLOCATION

The importance of hindfoot alignment should not be ignored. Feet are the foundation of the body. The alignment of the talus on the tarsal mechanism is the single most important determining factor that differentiates a rectus from malaligned hindfoot structure. The factor that differentiates normal from abnormal talotarsal alignment is the overlap of the articular facets (**Fig. 1**A). The talotarsal facets should always remain in constant congruent contact to be considered normal. Incongruent contact represents a dislocation deformity (see **Fig. 1**B). This partial dislocation (see **Fig. 1**C) leads to a pathologic chain reaction in the entire foot structure distally, and also proximally, up the musculoskeletal chain.[4] Symington,[5] in 1884, stated "it is at the talo-tarsal joint that the deformity commences, and it is here that the displacements occur that constitute its

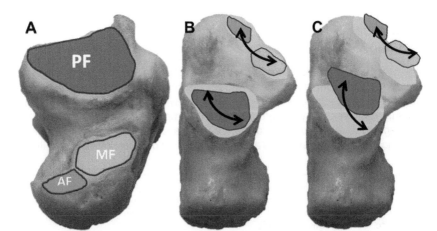

Fig. 1. (*A*) Plantar surface of the talus, highlighting the articular facets. The posterior facet (PF; *blue*), middle facet (MF; *yellow*), and anterior facet (AF; *green*) of the talus should remain in constant congruent contact with the counter facets on the calcaneus. (*B*) Counter facets on the calcaneus. (*C*) Partial dislocation of the joint. Note that the articular facets are incongruent.

most important features." This deformity may exist as a recurrent-dynamic/flexible, semireducible, or rigid-static/nonreducible condition. Clinically this is established via weight-bearing and non–weight-bearing examination. The recurrent-dynamic/flexible dislocation of the talus on the tarsal mechanism has a greater potential to contribute to secondary abnormalities than a rigid-static/nonreducible deformity. A flexible deformity is a dynamic malformation. While standing and with every step taken, excessive abnormal forces are acting on the osseous structures and soft tissues within the foot and ankle. A rigid foot has lost its "spring," and therefore does not have the same deforming forces transferred to the supporting tissues.

The partial dislocation of the talus on the tarsal mechanism allows for an abnormal transfer of forces from the body above. Forces that should be passing posterolaterally through the calcaneus are instead transferred anteromedially onto the medial column of the foot.[6] These excessive forces have to be compensated for by the ligaments stabilizing the talotarsal joint. When these ligaments fail to control the abnormal talotarsal motion caused by the osseous defect, an increased strain on the calcaneonavicular spring ligament results. Eventually the spring ligament may become compromised, because the calcaneus is forced posterolateral and the navicular is forced anteromedially.[7] Another common consequence of this partial dislocation is that navicular sag may occur from the direct impact forces from the head of the talus. The navicular is forced downward, producing a "fallen arch." When this occurs, the posterior tibialis tendon will experience increased strain as will the medial band of the plantar fascia.[6,8–11] This recurrent partial dislocation results in a pathologic gait with extending periods of pronation (overpronation or hyperpronation). Such deforming forces are reduced once the talotarsal joint is stabilized.

Talotarsal joint displacement is also the primary cause of the development of many forefoot disorders such as first-ray deformities, including hallux abductovalgus and limitus/rigidus, and flexor stabilization digital deformities.[12,13] As the talus displaces anteromedially, it causes a chain reaction of additional forces on these areas. Many surgical procedures are performed on these secondary deformities, yet rarely is the underlying etiology properly addressed, which could lead to a recurrence of those secondary deformities. Although the surgeon or clinician may have diagnosed the hindfoot deformity, in the author's opinion the treatment is often downplayed. With regard to the repair of a deformity, it is extremely important to identify the pathologic component(s) contributing to the overall deformity. Because the foot is the most complex dynamic mechanism of the body, it is important to observe concomitant structural defects. Identification of these angular deformities will provide a road map to the most successful solution. The angular relationships around the talotarsal joint must be evaluated. This region contains the most complex joint mechanism of the body, and arguably the most important in regard of weight-bearing activities. The talotarsal mechanism acts as a torque converter for forces both from the body above and from the ground below. If all of the other identified foot deformities are addressed yet the talotarsal joint remains malaligned, there will be suboptimal results and/or failure.

A stable and properly aligned foot structure is also very important when it comes to the proximal musculoskeletal chain. The talar alignment on the calcaneus determines the alignment to the knee.[14] The hip, pelvis, and lower back may also be affected by the partial talotarsal dislocation.[15,16] Often there are complaints of pain in these other areas, yet an evaluation of the mechanics of the foot is neglected when there no painful symptoms are reported. The failure of treatments to these areas is well documented. For example, studies have shown that 71% of all low back surgeries fail.[17] Failure is so common that there is even a diagnosis code (722.80) for "failed back surgery (post-laminectomy) syndrome."

Clinical Signs and Symptoms

It is fairly easy, even for an untrained observer, to recognize misaligned feet. Parents often can tell that something "just doesn't look right." There may or may not be a lowering of the natural arch of the foot. In many cases when there is no weight on the foot, there is a normal-appearing arch (**Fig. 2**A). However, on weight bearing the arch height decreases (see **Fig. 2**B), revealing the dynamic component to a flexible deformity compared with a rigid, nonflexible dislocation deformity.

The symptoms associated with a misaligned hindfoot structure can range dramatically. Some patients have no symptoms, or at least none in the foot and ankle. Others have significant activity-limiting pain, and some may even suffer psychological symptoms. Symptoms may not present initially on weight bearing but may set in after a period of weight bearing. A good example of post–weight-bearing pain is bedtime leg cramps, periostitis or "growing pains." Children who suffer from growing pains often have misaligned feet.[18] Talotarsal instability leads to a prolonged period of pronatory motion whereby the muscles in the leg have to work "harder" than they should, which leads to increased muscle pull and tension on the periosteum. This strain builds over the course of daily activity. Once the child is finally non–weight bearing when in bed, the tissues contract and the pain sets in. Parents often comment that the more active the child is throughout the day, the worse the pain is at night, and the less active the child is throughout the day the less pain there is at night, if any.[19]

When the child does not have a specific complaint of foot pain, there are other presenting clues that can be used as part of the clinical evaluation. A child with this deformity will not want to stand or walk for extended periods of time in comparison with someone with a normal hindfoot alignment. Children with misaligned feet are often less active than children with normal hindfoot alignment. Children with misaligned feet will usually run significantly slower than someone of the same age with a normal hindfoot alignment. If the child with a misaligned hindfoot is asked to stand, he or she will be unable to stand with equal weight on both feet without shifting the weight from one side of the body to the other.

There are even more nonconspicuous clues. Shoes can provide valuable information about the foot's alignment. First, there will be an uneven wear pattern. The outer part of the heel will be significantly worn. There could be a circular pattern under the metatarsal head area on the bottom of the shoe caused by an abnormal abductory twist. Even shoelaces becoming untied can be an indication of a malalignment of the foot, resulting from the repeated oblique force applied to the laces in place of anterior-posterior forces. Often the child will simply tuck the laces into the sides so they are not trampled on. Another indication that children are bothered by standing or walking is their complaining about or avoiding situations whereby prolonged

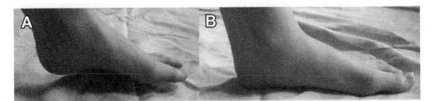

Fig. 2. (A) A non–weight-bearing foot with a normal arch, indicating that the talotarsal joint is properly aligned. (B) A weight-bearing foot in relaxed-stance position. The talus has partially dislocated on the tarsal mechanism, forcing the navicular to sag, which causes the partial collapse of the arch.

standing or walking is going to occur, and when it does there are repeated proclamations such as "can I sit down?" or "can we go now?"

Of course there are other indications of hindfoot misalignment, such as secondary deformities within the foot. The unnatural displacement and unlocking of the talotarsal joint leads to a dynamic chain reaction throughout the foot distally and proximally up the musculoskeletal system. Exactly where the symptoms ensue will be at the weakest link of the chain. Secondary findings such as first-ray deformities and flexor stabilization digital deformities may or may not be present. There may also be proximal symptoms to the knees, hips, and back.

The possibility that the deformity has not yet resulted in pain or secondary abnormalities, especially in children, is a primary factor in the differing opinions on treatment. Some physicians believe that the absence of pain means that damage is not occurring. Pain is an indication that something is wrong, an inherent warning signal. However, many times a pathologic deformity can be present without pain. With greater understanding of the larger and long-term implications of the failure to treat hindfoot instability, it should be easy to recognize that the absence of pain does not mean that treatment should not be initiated. There are many medical conditions that are treated without the presence of pain. The presence of pain and/or quality of life–limiting symptoms leads to a higher rate of acceptance of treatment, whereas the absence of pain or quality of life–limiting symptoms yields a lower chance of acceptance.

Furthermore, there are psychological symptoms that are almost always ignored and rarely considered important. Imagine the psychological toll to children when told that they are deformed. There are the ramifications of having to wear special shoes or inserts in shoes. Both of these have the impact of making children feel "different," or like they do not belong. There is an impact when they are not able to run as fast as their friends. Athletic prowess is an attribute that is highly valued in our culture. These children may have the desire to be active, but are punished with pain when they attempt physical activity.

EVALUATION

There have been many attempts to create a clinical standard to diagnose persons with flatfoot. Because of the many unique aspects of this disease entity, there are no clear delineating factors. Some look at arch height, heel valgus, and forefoot abduction. Many investigators have determined that the use of radiographs has proved to be the best diagnostic tool to establish a deformity.[20,21] While there has been commentary on many different aspects of the deformity, one primary factor has been consistent, namely the relationship of the talus to the rest of the foot bones—hence the word tal-i-pes.

An important part of the clinical examination is determining the flexibility of the dislocation deformity. A flexible deformity will have more treatment options than will a rigid condition. With a flexible deformity, the non–weight-bearing examination usually shows a normal-appearing arch. On weight bearing there is lowering of the arch. The weight-bearing comparison of relaxed-stance with neutral-stance positions establishes the reducibility of this deformity (**Fig. 3**). This maneuver shows the parent where the child's foot should be (correct position) and where the foot is in reality (incorrect position).

The author believes that it is difficult to test for a true equinus deformity in a pediatric patient, owing to the natural guarding mechanism of the Achilles-gastrosoleal complex. An abrupt dorsiflexion of the foot triggers a tendon reflex that signals the triceps surae to plantarflex in reaction to such a stimulus. Often a child who is thought to have a tight Achilles tendon is brought to the operating room for a lengthening procedure.

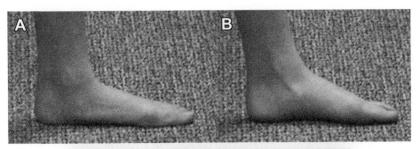

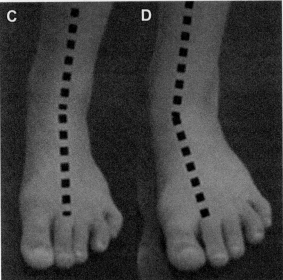

Fig. 3. (*A*) Medial view of a weight-bearing foot and ankle with the talotarsal joint in neutral position. (*B*) Same view with the patient in relaxed-stance position. (*C*) Anterior view of the foot and ankle of another individual with the talotarsal joint in neutral position. (*D*) Same foot and view in relaxed-stance position. In both comparisons, the neutral view shows the talus aligned on the calcaneus, and the relaxed-stance view shows the talus partially dislocated on the calcaneus.

Once the general anesthesia is administered and the reflex eliminated, no equinus deformity is found.

A gait analysis will often reveal the "too many toes" sign or abducted gait and abductory twist. A look at heel lift is also important to show the function of the Achilles. Some children compensate for a partial talotarsal dislocation by walking on the tips of their toes. This toe-walking maintains the articular facets of the talotarsal joint and maintains the efficiency of the tendo Achilles and posterior tibial tendon. It is important to check for a metatarsus adductus component of this deformity, as a skewfoot could be present. In a rigid deformity, one should suspect a tarsal coalition.

RADIOGRAPHIC FEATURES

Radiographic evaluation is an extremely useful tool in confirming a suspicion of deformity. An even more valuable tool is the use of weight-bearing fluoroscopy. The ability to dynamically observe the internal osseous interactions is far superior to a "snapshot in time." Not only does fluoroscopy provide the clinician with detailed data on range of motion, it provides an outstanding educational tool for the patient. Imagine trying to explain talotarsal range of motion to patients rather than actually showing them the motion.

When dynamic fluoroscopy is not available, it is highly recommended to obtain 2 sets of weight-bearing radiographs. The first are the traditional view with the feet in relaxed/natural stance, and the second is with the child's foot placed in neutral position. These comparative studies provide many diagnostic clues. First, they help to establish the degree of deformity via objective comparative angular measurements. Second, they establish the flexibility or reducibility of the deformity that will guide treatment options. Finally, they help as an educational tool to explain the deformity to the parents and child.

There are specific landmarks to be evaluated. On the lateral radiographs, a comparison of neutral with relaxed stance will show 1 or more of the following signs, depending on the planar dominance (if any) of the deformity: an open versus obliterated sinus tarsi, an increase in the talar declination angle (>21°), an anterior deviation of the cyma line, an increase in the talar first metatarsal angle, a decrease in the calcaneal inclination angle, and navicular drop (**Fig. 4**). On the anteroposterior view, the talar second metatarsal angle provides the easiest and most effective tool to evaluate the relationship between the hindfoot and forefoot. An increase in this angle signifies a transverse plane deformity (>16°). The clinician must always look for the radiographic signs of a tarsal coalition such as the "halo sign," "comma sign," or "anteater nose sign." If suspicion exists, then further studies such as computed tomography or magnetic resonance imaging should be prescribed.

CONSERVATIVE TREATMENT

The nonsurgical management of misaligned feet is usually the treatment option of choice. However, a critical analysis reveals a major flaw. The pathologic osseous deformity does not self-correct. There is no evidence that a child's foot self-corrects with time. True pathologic conditions will either remain the same or become progressively worse. An acute trauma may respond well to conservative care, but this congenital deformity will not. This deformity is an internal one that requires internal correction, at least if more than the temporary alleviation of symptoms is expected.

Osgood,[22] in his treatise on the treatment of faulty weight bearing, provided 5 conclusions:

1. That a rigid arch supporter worn for several months, while relieving symptoms in the majority of cases, weakens the foot and tends to make the wearer dependent on it.
2. That the prolonged use of such rigid supports is, in the great majority of cases, unnecessary, if proper treatment is administered at the appropriate time.
3. That the aim of the surgeon should be to strengthen the weak structure, and not to temporarily relieve symptoms.
4. That in the cases of weak foot the talocalcaneal articulation demands most attention.
5. That in severe cases of long standing, operative measures may be more commonly used and offer lasting relief.

One form of conservative care is to attempt to strengthen the weakened muscles that are failing to support the foot. The theory that there is a failure of the soft tissues is not in fact the situation in most cases. The talus has no tendon insertion. Its motion is

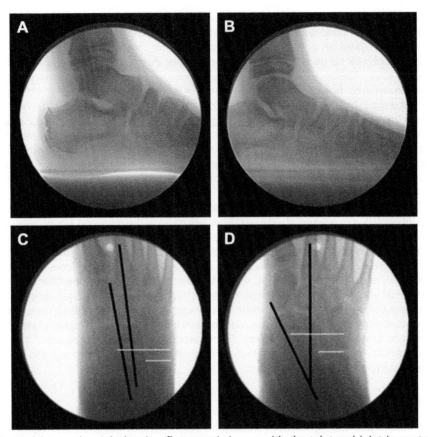

Fig. 4. (*A*) Lateral weight-bearing fluoroscopic image with the talotarsal joint in neutral position. Note the open sinus tarsi and the position of the navicular in comparison with the cuboid. The articular facets are in congruent contact. (*B*) Same patient in relaxed-stance position. The talus has partially dislocated anteriorly, inducing a sagittal plane deformity. Note the obliteration of the sinus tarsi, navicular drop, and increased talar declination angle. There is minimal change to the calcaneal inclination angle. (*C*) Anteroposterior weight-bearing fluoroscopic image with the talotarsal joint in neutral position. Note that the talar second metatarsal angle is less than 16°. (*D*) Same patient, weight bearing with the foot in relaxed-stance position. Note that the talar second metatarsal angle is greater than 16°, indicating a transverse plane deformity. There is also an anterior component; the anterior edge of the talus is more distal in comparison with the anterior edge of the calcaneus.

far more influenced by the articular facets than by the ligamentous attachments. The pronator muscles are already contracting, and increased strain is placed on the tendons. These musculotendinous units are on high alert to prevent the excessive pronatory movement of the talotarsal joint.[10] Therefore to say that the child needs to strengthen these muscles even more is simply unrealistic.

The use of prefabricated or custom-fabricated orthoses in the treatment of talotarsal displacement remains very questionable.[23] These plantar "arch-support" devices only play a supportive, not corrective or curative, role.[24] These devices, placed under the foot, are supposed to stabilize structures above the bottom of the foot. It does not make much sense that a device placed below the calcaneus could control the excessive talar motion occurring above the calcaneus. Many are led to believe that a cure will occur if the child wears the device long enough, but this has not been established.

It has been established that symptoms can vary and that pain is not always present. Therefore, symptom relief would be a poor method of evaluating the effectiveness of the treatment chosen. Although symptom relief is something that is sought it cannot, by itself, prove results. Radiographic evidence is used to prove the presence of the deformity; therefore, it makes sense to use radiographic evidence to prove the efficacy of the treatment in realigning the talotarsal joint. Indeed this is the standard protocol for surgical procedures, to compare preprocedure radiographs with postprocedure radiographs. One reason why radiographs are not taken with conservative treatment is simply because they have consistently failed to show any significant amount of osseous realignment (**Fig. 5**).[23]

Although it may seem that the use of an orthosis falls in line with the philosophy of "do no harm," it does not pass any litmus tests. There is no evidence showing significant control of the excessive talotarsal motion, meaning that while standing, walking, or running, excessive forces continue to act on the structures within the foot distally and also proximally, affecting the ankle, knee, hip, and, possibly, the back. Meanwhile, the child and parents are under the impression that the device is actually "fixing" the problem, which is simply not true. There is a false sense of "correction." Several studies have been undertaken that have been unable to provide the necessary evidence for the efficacy of nonsurgical interventions for children with flexible flat feet.[25] Although it has not been established that an orthosis can control or correct talotarsal motion, it can potentially assist in rebalancing the center line of gravity passing through the rest of the foot. There is a role for the use of orthoses, but their effectiveness in controlling the most important aspect of this deformity has not been established.

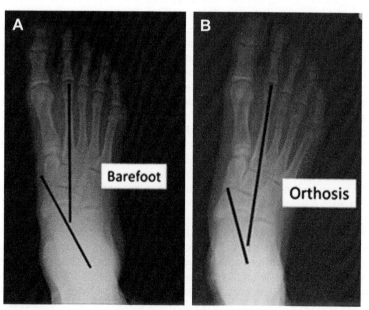

Fig. 5. (*A*) Relaxed-stance anteroposterior view of a foot showing a significant transverse plane deformity. (*B*) Same foot, also in relaxed stance, weight bearing on a custom-fit orthosis. Note that the transverse plane deformity is still present.

SURGICAL OPTIONS

The goal of musculoskeletal surgery is to realign malaligned structures and to maintain the alignment with the least harm to the adjacent structures. A benefit-risk analysis must be considered before any surgical procedure because there are no complication-free operations. Moreover, when it comes to the repair of a deformity it should be realized by the patient that no matter how talented the surgeon, it is impossible to completely and perfectly repair the deformity. Consider a bent paperclip; it can never be bent back to its exact original shape.

Attention must be directed to the apex of the deformity. The first place that must be corrected is the partial dislocation of the talus on the tarsal mechanism. The stability of the talotarsal joint has to be reestablished so that the articular facets remain in constant congruent contact. This accomplishment, by itself, immediately redistributes the joint forces and decreases the excessive strain to the supporting soft tissues.[6,8,9,26–29]

Attempts to correct talotarsal displacement through alterations of the calcaneus, whether through a posterior medial slide or anterior bone grafting, do little to stabilize the excessive talar motion.[30] Historically arthrodesis procedures were advocated, until long-term follow-up revealed an alarming rate of arthritic changes to the proximal and distal joints.[31] Various osseous and soft-tissue procedures have been encouraged and later discouraged, because of the associated complications.[32] Most times the presenting deformity did not severely limit the patient, which could be the end result of a too aggressive surgical stabilization.

An inventive change in thinking to develop a less invasive technique to stabilize the talus through the use of a joint-blocking/limiting implement began with Chambers.[33] There has since been an evolution of materials and device designs that has produced very encouraging results.[34] Many foot and ankle surgeons choose extraosseous talotarsal stabilization (EOTTS) devices, while there are still those foot and ankle surgeons who use an intraosseous arthroereisis device.

The use of a joint-sparing, less invasive, yet more dynamic technique that redirects muscle forces and diminishes the morbidity and risk of complications associated with reconstruction, without compromising the outcome, should be favored over a joint-destroying technique. Surgeons should follow the "less is more" motto when considering surgical options, when indicated. Literature has shown that the use of an EOTTS device is both safer and more effective, especially in comparison with traditional techniques and their associated complications.[35] There is a preponderance of evidence showing the benefit of an EOTTS procedure to decrease strain to the medial band of the plantar fascia, posterior tibial tendon, and tibial posterior nerve, and to decrease pressures within both the tarsal tunnel and porta pedis.[8,9,26,27]

Radiographically, EOTTS has been shown to reduce the amount of sagittal plane sag of the navicular[28] and correct both transverse and sagittal plane talotarsal deformities (**Fig. 6**).[29] A limitation of EOTTS is that it has not been shown to have an effect on the calcaneal inclination angle, either positively or negatively. Therefore, if the patient has a lower than normal calcaneal inclination angle, other surgical procedures, such as gastrosoleal lengthening or a calcaneal osteotomy, should be considered.

Why not use a more conservative, "reversible" procedure before a more "aggressive" procedure? A subtalar implant "leaves the door open"; if that option fails, the next level of surgical procedures can be attempted. The more advanced surgical options may provide a more definitive result, but at a much higher possibility of complication and without the reversibility factor. Many studies have analyzed these techniques, and have provided various conclusions. A recent study[30] compared medial

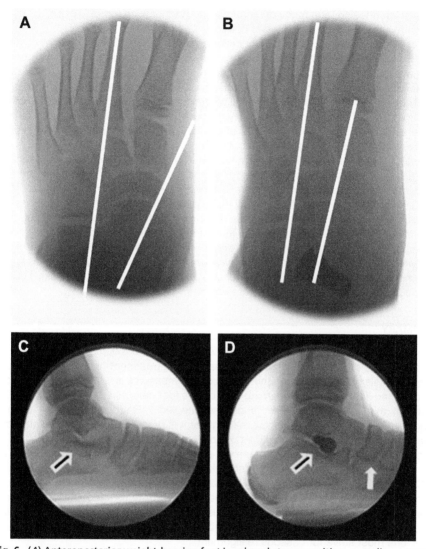

Fig. 6. (*A*) Anteroposterior weight-bearing foot in relaxed-stance position, revealing a transverse plane deformity. (*B*) Post-extraosseous talotarsal stabilization with normalization of the talar second metatarsal angle. (*C*) Lateral weight-bearing foot in relaxed-stance position. There is obliteration of the sinus tarsi, and evidence of a sagittal plane deformity, including an increase in the talar declination angle, navicular sag, and plantarflexion of the sustentaculum tali, as is seen in its opacity within the calcaneus (*open arrow*). (*D*) Same foot and view in weight-bearing relaxed-stance post-extraosseous talotarsal stabilization. Note the normalization of the talar declination angle, restoration of the navicular height (*closed arrow*), and the disappearance of the sustentaculum tali opacity (*open arrow*).

translational osteotomy of the calcaneus and lateral column lengthening in combination with flexor digitorum longus to the midfoot in adults. The results showed that lateral column lengthening was more corrective than medialization of the calcaneus; however, there was a higher rate of arthritis in the adjacent joints with the lateral column lengthening, and many other complications including removal of painful internal hardware, nonunion, and loss of correction.

Many patients also have naviculocuneiform vaulting or instability at the naviculocuneiform joint or first metatarsocuneiform joint. Failure to stabilize these joints could compromise the result of an EOTTS procedure. It is possible that once the deforming posterior forces are reduced, these distal joints will self-correct; however, this depends on both the severity and flexibility of those concurrent deformities. The combination of EOTTS with an orthosis may be beneficial and worth the attempt before more surgery to stabilize the joints is attempted. A severe or rigid deformity would not respond to this less aggressive approach.

Finally, a coexisting equinus deformity may also be present. Many have theorized that an equinus deformity contributes to hindfoot abnormality,[36,37] and a lengthening procedure should be performed if there is a failure in conservative measures, such as stretching, to lengthen the tendon. Although lengthening the tendon can increase a calcaneal inclination angle that is lower than normal, there are no data to suggest normalization of the talotarsal joint via lengthening of the tendo Achilles. It has been the author's experience that many mild and moderate forms of equinus have resolved following an EOTTS procedure. In severe cases of equinus, a surgical release could be recommended in the same surgical setting as an EOTTS procedure, whereas it could be staged in cases of mild to moderate equinus.

SUMMARY

The ability to differentiate between a somewhat simple and a complex deformity provides valuable decision-making factors regarding the treatment of foot abnormalities. The emphasis toward internal rather than external measures is warranted. Most pediatricians' advice to parents regarding their child's foot deformity is to simply ignore it, although this really amounts to "supervised neglect." Flatfoot deformities do not magically self-correct. A pathologic malalignment is present, which requires physical intervention. The displacement of the talus on the calcaneus and navicular is not a life-threatening disease, but does represent a powerful dynamic deformity that leads to destruction not only within the foot and ankle but also up the musculoskeletal chain.

Conservative options seem to do little harm and may help to decrease short-term pain. However, published studies have shown an inability to adequately realign the internal osseous structures. Therefore, a false sense of correction is given to patients, amounting to almost a placebo effect. Although not every patient is a surgical candidate, one must strive for osseous realignment.

When conservative options fail to provide adequate symptom relief or inadequately address the underlying deformity, internal correction should be considered. The first step requires the restoration of the talotarsal joint alignment. The reason why many physicians stress conservative care over surgical procedures is due to the seemingly radical techniques required to reconstruct the foot's alignment. For this reason it is important to recognize the true etiology of the malalignment, which is discovered by comparison of weight-bearing radiographs. When the deformity is shown to be flexible, there is no reason not to proceed with less aggressive techniques such as extraosseous talotarsal stabilization because "no bridges are burned." If there is a failure of EOTTS, the device can be removed and more advanced surgical procedures can be attempted: the "less is more" approach.

The deformity, for some patients, is so complex that other surgical procedures at multiple sites are required. Sometimes surgical correction may need to wait until the child reaches adulthood. In other cases, it may be that the simple insertion of an

EOTTS device will realign the talotarsal joint and therefore eliminate the most important deforming forces—the sooner, the better.

The author submits that adult-acquired flatfoot, which is a symptomatic posterior tibial tendon, is often the result of years of leaving this pediatric deformity untreated. These adults did not have a "normal" alignment yesterday and then got of bed today only to watch their foot collapse. Rather, the decades of standing, walking, or running with a malaligned foot led to the eventual strain and partial rupture of the posterior tibial tendon. Consider the fact that the average person takes nearly 7000 steps a day, which multiplied over 45 years equals nearly 116 million times the posterior tibial tendon was overstretched. If the talus would have been internally stabilized this strain would have been reduced, therefore likely preventing this complication.

The financial impact of this disease entity must also be considered. In 2008, in the United States there were 62 million adults who reported back pain and another 39 million who complained of knee pain.[38] The direct cost of musculoskeletal disorders was $575 million. Adding the indirect costs resulted in $950 million. It seems that there are no final cures to knee, hip, or back pain. One wonders how many of these people were told that their misaligned feet were of no concern, and who as a child were told that nothing needed to be done; now after tens of millions of steps the repetitive damage has destroyed their knees, hips, and back. One wonders how their lives would have been positively affected by the use of an effective internal intervention. A misaligned pediatric foot must not be ignored or shrugged off as normal. This condition will potentially lead to devastating musculoskeletal effects. In the majority of cases, the benefits of the surgical procedure far outweigh the potential risks.

REFERENCES

1. Whitman R. The treatment of flat feet. J Bone Joint Surg 01;s1–1(1):122–137, 1889.
2. American Academy of Pediatrics. Flat feet and fallen arches. http://www.healthychildren.org/English/health-issues/conditions/orthopedic/pages/Flat-Feet-Fallen-Arches.aspx?nfstatus=401&nftoken=00000000-0000-0000-0000-000000000000&nfstatusdescription=ERROR%3a+No+local+token. Accessed July 29, 2013.
3. Mosca VS. Flexible flatfoot in children and adolescents. J Child Orthop 2010;4: 107–21.
4. Friedman MA, Draganich LF, Toolan B, et al. The effects of adult acquired flatfoot deformity on tibiotalar joint contact characteristics. Foot Ankle Int 2001;22(3): 241–6.
5. Symington J. The anatomy of acquired flat-foot. J Anat Physiol 1884;19(Pt 1): 82.2–3.
6. Graham ME, Parikh R, Goel V, et al. Stabilization of joint forces of the subtalar complex via Hyprocure sinus tarsi stent. J Am Podiatr Med Assoc 2011;101(5): 390–9.
7. Williams BR, Ellis SJ, Deyer TW, et al. Reconstruction of the spring ligament using a peroneus longus autograft tendon transfer. Foot Ankle Int 2010;31:567–77.
8. Graham ME, Jawrani N, Goel V. Evaluation plantar fascia strain in hyperpronating cadaveric feet following an extra-osseous talotarsal stabilization procedure. J Foot Ankle Surg 2011;50(6):682–6.
9. Graham ME, Jawrani N, Goel V. Effect of extra-osseous talotarsal stabilization on posterior tibial tendon strain in hyperpronating feet. J Foot Ankle Surg 2011;50(6): 672–5.

10. Lapidus PW. Spastic flat-foot. J Bone Joint Surg Am 1946;28(1):126–36.

11. Cornwall MW, McPoil TG. Plantar fasciitis: etiology and treatment. J Orthop Sports Phys Ther 1999;29(12):756–60.

12. Eustace S. Hallux valgus, first metatarsal pronation and collapse of the medial longitudinal arch–a radiological correlation. Skeletal Radiol 1994;23(3):191–4.

13. Kalen V, Brecher A. Relationship between adolescent bunions and flatfeet. Foot Ankle Int 1988;8(6):331–6.

14. Levinger P, Menz HB, Rotoohabad MR, et al. Foot posture in people with medial compartment knee osteoarthritis. J Foot Ankle Res 2010;3:29.

15. Nguyen AD, Shultz SJ. Identifying relationships among lower extremity alignment characteristics. J Athl Train 2009;44(5):511–8.

16. Khamis S, Yizhar Z. Effect of feet hyperpronation on pelvic alignment in a standing position. Gait Posture 2007;25:127–34.

17. Dananberg HJ, Guiliano M. Chronic low back pain and its response to custom foot orthoses. J Am Podiatr Med Assoc 1999;89(3):109–17.

18. Brenning R. Growing pain. Acta Soc Med Ups 1960;65:185–201.

19. Evans A, Scutter S, Lang L, et al. 'Growing pains' in young children: a study of the profile, experiences and quality of life issues of four to six year old children with recurrent leg pain. J Foot Ankle Res 2006;16:120–4.

20. Staheli LT. Planovalgus foot deformity—current status. J Am Podiatr Med Assoc 1999;89(2):94–9.

21. Benedetti MG, Berti L, Straudi S, et al. Clinicoradiographic assessment of flexible flatfoot in children. J Am Podiatr Med Assoc 2010;100(6):463–71.

22. Osgood RB. The treatment of faulty weight-bearing in "weak" and "flat" feet. J Bone Joint Surg Am 1906;s2-4(2):137–49.

23. Bordelon RL. Correction of hypermobile flatfoot in children by molded insert. Foot Ankle Int 1980;1(3):143–50.

24. Penneua K, Lutter LD, Winter RD. Pes planus: radiographic changes with foot orthoses and shoes. Foot Ankle Int 1982;2(5):299–303.

25. Mackenzie J, Rome K, Evans AM. The efficacy of nonsurgical interventions for pediatric flexible flat foot: a critical review. J Pediatr Orthop 2012;32(8):830–4.

26. Graham ME, Jawrani N, Goel V. The effect of extra-osseous talotarsal stabilization on posterior tibial nerve strain in hyperpronating feet: a cadaveric evaluation. J Foot Ankle Surg 2011;50(6):676–81.

27. Graham ME, Jawrani N, Goel V. The effect of hyprocure sinus tarsi stent on tarsal tunnel compartment pressures in hyperpronating feet. J Foot Ankle Surg 2011; 50(1):40–9.

28. Graham ME, Jawrani NT, Chikka A. Radiographic evaluation of navicular position in the sagittal plane -correction following extra-osseous talotarsal stabilization. J Foot Ankle Surg 2011;50(5):551–7.

29. Graham ME, Jawrani NT, Chikka A, et al. Surgical treatment of hyperpronation using an extraosseous talotarsal stabilization device: radiographic outcomes in 70 adult patients. J Foot Ankle Surg 2012;51(5):548–55.

30. Bolt PM, Coy S, Toolan BC. A comparison of lateral column lengthening and medial translational osteotomy of the calcaneus for the reconstruction of adult acquired flatfoot. Foot Ankle Int 2007;28(11):1115–23.

31. Crego C, Ford L. An end result study of various procedures for correcting flatfeet in children. J Bone Joint Surg Am 1952;34(1):183–95.

32. Sekiya JK, Saltman CL. Long term follow-up of medial column fusion and tibialis anterior transposition for adolescent flatfoot deformity. Iowa Orthop J 1997;17: 121–9.

33. Chambers EF. An operation for the correction of flexible flat feet of adolescents. West J Surg Obstet Gynecol 1946;54(3):77–86.

34. Graham ME, Jawrani NT, Chikka A. Extra-osseous talotarsal stabilization using hyprocure in adults: a 5-year retrospective follow-up. J Foot Ankle Surg 2012; 51(1):23–9.

35. Metcalfe SA, Bowling FL, Reeves ND. Subtalar joint arthroereisis in the management of pediatric flexible flatfoot: a critical review of literature. Foot Ankle Int 2011; 32(12):1127–39.

36. Grady JF, Kelly C. Endoscopic gastrocnemius recession for treating equinus in pediatric patients. Clin Orthop Relat Res 2010;468(4):1033–8.

37. Meszaros A, Caudell G. The surgical management of equinus in the adult acquired flatfoot. Clin Podiatr Med Surg 2007;24(4):667–85.

38. Agency for Healthcare Research and Quality: Medical Expenditure Panel Survey. Statistical brief #331, p. 1–5, 2011.

Principles of Management of Growth Plate Fractures in the Foot and Ankle

Paul Dayton, DPM, MS, FACFAS[a],*, Mindi Feilmeier, DPM, FACFAS[b],
Nathan Coleman, DPM[a]

KEYWORDS

- Pediatric fracture • Growth plate injury • Physis fracture • Salter Harris

KEY POINTS

- Physeal injuries are an interesting and challenging group of injuries based on the unique characteristics of skeletally immature bone and the developing pediatric patient.
- Providers who treat pediatric injuries must have a detailed understanding of not only the histologic and mechanical properties of the pediatric skeleton, but also understand and be sensitive to the psychological and social expectations of the patients and their families.
- The provider is challenged to meet the expectations for communication regarding not only the immediate needs of the injured patient, but also the long-term prognosis of the injury.
- Clearly stated goals and limitations of treatments must be given by the provider to gain the trust and compliance of the patient and his or her family. Detailed understanding of the fracture mechanism and fracture patterns is essential for accurate diagnosis and treatment.
- The provider must constantly remain vigilant for expected and unexpected changes in the osseous and soft tissue structures during treatment.
- Failure to recognize signs of growth interruption and progressive changes in position during healing or subsequent years of growth may lead to devastating functional abnormalities.

UNIQUE BONE QUALITIES OF THE PEDIATRIC SKELETON

Understanding the histologic make up of pediatric bone and how this relates to mechanical and healing properties is the starting point in evaluation and management of pediatric fractures. Histologically, woven bone predominates in the skeletally immature patient. Mechanically, woven bone responds differently to external stress than

[a] Trinity Regional Medical Center, UnityPoint Foot & Ankle, 804 Kenyon Road, Suite 310, Fort Dodge, IA 50501, USA; [b] College of Podiatric Medicine & Surgery, Des Moines University, 3200 Grand Avenue, Des Moines, IA 50312, USA
* Corresponding author.
E-mail address: daytonp@me.com

Clin Podiatr Med Surg 30 (2013) 583–598
http://dx.doi.org/10.1016/j.cpm.2013.07.004
0891-8422/13/$ – see front matter © 2013 Elsevier Inc. All rights reserved.

podiatric.theclinics.com

compact or lamellar bone found in the mature skeleton. In order to accurately diagnose and manage these fractures, it is imperative that the physician understands the skeletal age of the patient. Certain fracture patterns predominate at various stages of development, and clinical decisions are sometimes based as much on the stage of development as on the fracture pattern. Structurally, woven bone is more porous than lamellar bone. However, the mineral ratio of pediatric bone is the same as compact bone. The ratio of woven bone to compact bone changes during development. Mechanically, pediatric bone has increased capacity for plastic deformation and decreased tendency for comminution when compared with adult bone. When a mechanical stress is placed on the bone, the tendency is to fail in response to compression forces more often than with tension forces. This compression force can result in an incomplete fracture from plastic deformation known as a Torus or buckle fracture. These injuries are commonly seen in children at multiple ages. Another type of incomplete fracture based on the plastic properties of pediatric bone is the greenstick fracture. Unlike the torus fracture, a greenstick has an incomplete fracture on the tension side of the bone. Unless significantly displaced, treatment of a Torus or Greenstick fracture requires only support in a cast or a brace, as these fractures are usually stable. Healing times are usually short, and complications are rare (**Fig. 1**).

The periosteum of pediatric bone is thicker and more robust than in the adult skeleton. It is loosely attached at the diaphysis and tightly adhered to the metaphyseal cortex and the epiphyseal perichondrium. In addition, the periosteal tissues and ligaments are stronger than the adjacent physis and woven bone. Because of these properties, in many pediatric fractures, the periosteal tissues remain intact after fracture. This is important for healing of the fracture; additionally, it can aid in reduction of fractures by providing a tether to hold the fragments in alignment during traction maneuvers used in closed reduction.

Pediatric bone and the periosteum are very vascular and extremely osteogenic, allowing rapid healing. The vascular supply to pediatric bone arrives from multiple sources. Epiphyseal bone blood supply is derived from capsular soft tissue attachments and nutrient arteries that enter the epiphysis and supply both the epiphysis and the germinal layer of the physis. Metaphyseal vascular supply is mainly from endosteal vessels that form capillary loops. These arteries provide vascularization to the portion actively undergoing ossification but do not provide flow to the distal physis. The physis gets its vascular supply from epiphyseal, metaphyseal, and perichondral contributions. It is also important to understand that epiphyseal and metaphyseal blood supplies remain distinct with no vascular interconnection crossing the physis. As in the adult skeleton, the articular cartilage has no independent blood supply. Articular cartilage receives its nutrition from synovial fluid. Cartilage viability is dependent on synovial fluid production and distribution. Fluid production is dependent on active and passive joint motion. Joint motion signals synovial fluid production and also distributes the fluid, and is therefore vital to articular health and preservation of articular anatomy and function. Every attempt should be made to maintain passive and/or active joint motion during recovery. Stable fixation provides a platform for early range of motion and early rehabilitation. Conversely, excessively long periods of casting and immobilization are detrimental to joint health and should be avoided.

PHYSEAL HISTOLOGY

The physis is made up of 3 zones, with multiple layers residing in each zone. The zone nearest the epiphysis is the growth zone made up of the germinal and proliferative layers. This zone is responsible for the longitudinal growth of the bone as cells

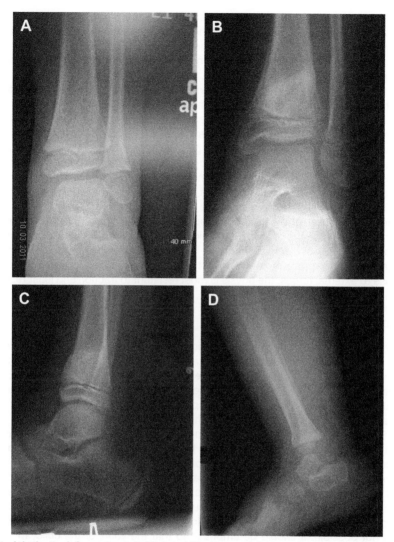

Fig. 1. (*A*) Plastic deformation of tibial and fibular metaphysis. Failure has occurred at the compression side of the bone, designating this as a torus fracture. Minimal displacement of this fracture is noted. Casting is the treatment of choice, and growth interruption is unlikely. (*B, C*) Typical radiographic findings on anterior-posterior (AP) and lateral views during healing of torus fracture of the tibia in an adolescent. (*D*) Buckle or torus fracture of the distal tibia in a young patient. Plastic deformation with minimal displacement requires no reduction. The displacement in this case is minimal and is in the plane of joint motion and therefore should be well tolerated.

move from a resting state in the germinal layer to an area of rapid mitosis and division in the proliferative layer, or layer of columniation.

The second zone is the zone of cartilage maturation, in which resides the hypertrophic layer and layer of calcification. This zone is largely composed of chondrocytes, which enlarge significantly in the hypertrophic layer, disintegrate, and then form a layer of necrotic calcified cells that develop a network of tunnels for the infiltration of osteoblasts and metaphyseal vessels. This zone is the weakest area of the physis and is especially susceptible to shearing, bending, and tension forces. Although this is known to be the weakest zone, it has been noted that 50% of physeal injuries cross multiple zones.

The final zone of ossification or transformation has 2 layers and is closest to the metaphysis. The layers are divided into the layer of vascular penetration and zone of ossification. In these layers, metaphyseal vessels penetrate the layer of calcified chondrocytes. This is followed by osteoblastic activity and subsequent osteogenesis.[1]

The zone of Ranvier is a circumferential groove that surrounds the periphery of the physis. This zone consists of prechondrocytes as well as fibroblasts and fibrocytes. The osseous ring of Lacroix is an extension of the metaphyseal cortex that is present within this zone. This area aids in support of the physis at the weak osteochondral junction and aids in securing the epiphysis to the metaphysis.

As noted previously, physeal vascular supply is from 3 sources, and the vessels are not connected across the physis. Mechanically, physeal tissue is weaker than metaphyseal, epiphyseal, or diaphyseal bone. It is also significantly weaker than ligaments; the ligaments are approximately 2 to 5 times stronger than the growth plate. In response to external forces, the physis is most resistant to traction and least resistant to torsion.

REMODELING

Due to the constantly changing state of pediatric bone, remodeling of a fracture can occur during the remaining period of growth. Limited osseous adaptation and improvement in position and function are possible. In some circumstances, less than perfect anatomic reduction in the acute setting may be acceptable. For example, angulation of long bone fractures may improve over time secondary to input from external forces. There are limitations to this concept however; angulation of more than 15° is not acceptable, and as the angulation approaches 90° to the plane of motion of the segment, remodeling is less likely. Additionally, if a displaced fracture crosses the physis at 90°, remodeling is not likely.

There are circumstances in which remodeling will not occur. Intra-articular fractures should be accurately reduced in all cases. Acute shortening will not improve with growth and development. Shortening should always be addressed during initial or subsequent reduction attempts. Axial rotation is also a circumstance in which remodeling is not possible. It should be emphasized that the younger the child, the more likely remodeling is to occur. If the child has less than 1 to 2 years of growth remaining, remodeling should not be relied upon, and the physician should obtain accurate reduction.

PHYSEAL INJURY MANAGEMENT

Before deciding on a course of treatment and before making recommendations regarding care of a pediatric patient, a detailed evaluation of the patient with thorough history and physical examination should done. Medical conditions along with associated vascular, neurologic, rheumatologic, and soft tissue concerns must be addressed in the treatment plan. Next, radiographic examination should be focused on the injured anatomic zone and any possible associated injuries. For extremity trauma, a minimum of 3 planar views should be obtained. Complicated or intra-articular fractures should be evaluated with computed tomography (CT) scans with additional multiplanar reconstructions. Comparison radiographs of the uninjured extremity can be very useful to determine normal anatomy and pick up subtle fractures or dislocations. Stress views are needed in certain injuries that carry expected instability. When evaluation of the patient and fracture injury has been assessed, closed reduction is typically attempted with consent from the patient and family to proceed to open reduction if closed reduction is not possible. There are certain fractures in which closed reduction is not practical or possible. In these cases, primary open reduction internal fixation (ORIF) should be chosen and unnecessary closed reduction attempts avoided. If a fracture cannot be maintained with splintage, such as with distal forefoot fractures, attempts at reduction should be avoided to prevent further damage to the growth plate and associated structures. Similarly, if a reasonable attempt at closed reduction fails, multiple attempts at forced closed reduction should be avoided to prevent further injury.

Both closed reductions and open reductions need to be performed with a measured amount of force to prevent further damage to the physis that could result in destruction of the germinal layers. With closed reduction, more focus should be placed on traction rather than forceful manipulation of the fracture fragments. Due to the robust nature of the pediatric periosteum, ligamentotaxis many times will produce anatomic reduction. For closed reductions, the patient should be sedated or anesthetized to prevent pain and provide relaxation of the extremity. Muscle spasm and tense muscle compartments will prevent reduction and will make appropriate casting extremely difficult. Radiographs should be repeated immediately after reduction and at intervals during recovery to ensure adequate reduction is maintained.

Surgical principles begin with careful tissue handling and dissection technique to preserve blood supply. Priority should be given to indirect reduction techniques and percutaneous fixation when possible. During ORIF, every effort should be made to limit growth center damage with overzealous exposure and tissue stripping. For instance, the surgeon should not disturb the physeal periosteum and peri-fracture soft tissues. Principles of physeal injury fixation focus on prevention of further damage to the physis and growth interruption. When necessary, pins can be temporarily placed across the physis to engage and stabilize epiphyseal or metaphyseal fractures. However, only smooth pins should cross the physis, and these should be removed as soon as practical. Additionally, parallel pins are safer than crossed pins, and screws or other fixation techniques producing compression should not traverse the physis. Repeat radiographic examination should take place every 6 to 12 months after fracture healing until growth is completed to assess for any growth disturbances.

CASE STUDIES

The most utilized classification system used in pediatric fractures is the Salter-Harris classification. There are 5 types originally noted, which are based on the location of the fracture or fractures distal and proximal to the physis. There are further subgroups that have been added to the original classification system, which describe unique circumstances. Understanding of this classification system is very helpful in determining proper treatment and assessing long-term prognosis.

Type 1

This fracture pattern is defined by a slip through the physis only and tends to occur in younger children. Because of its strength, the periosteal hinge usually remains intact. These fractures have a good prognosis for healing and a low incidence of epiphysiodesis. Keep in mind that these fractures may not be visible on radiograph; therefore, a high degree of clinical suspicion and a thorough physical examination are important.[2]

Treatment consists of closed reduction if displaced and splintage with a cast or brace. In the first 3 weeks, weight-bearing status is determined based on the fracture site and propensity for displacement. Once clinical signs of recovery including decreased pain and improved range of motion are noted, the patient can be transitioned to a weight-bearing cast or walking boot for an additional 3 weeks. Radiographic findings such as fracture gap filling and extensive callus may signal physeal growth interruption. Healing is usually rapid, especially in younger patients, and growth interruption is typically unlikely in this injury pattern (**Figs. 2** and **3**).

Type 2

This fracture pattern is the most common physeal injury. In this group, a transverse slip of the physis, along with a fracture through the metaphysis, is evident. This fracture pattern is more commonly seen in children over 10 years of age.[3] If stable and not significantly displaced, this injury may be treated with closed reduction with external splinting. Prognosis for healing is good, with a low incidence of growth interruption. Significantly displaced fractures that cannot be closed reduced or that remain unstable following reduction require fixation. The importance of careful handling of the soft tissues and gentle reduction techniques can not be overemphasized to prevent further

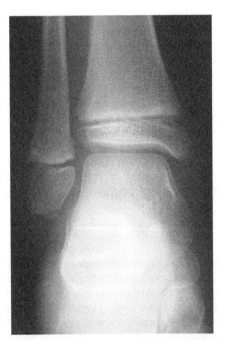

Fig. 2. Type 1 injury of the distal fibular physis. The displacement within the physis is subtle, and there is no fracture of the epiphysis or metaphysis. Clinical examination is extremely important for diagnosis. Treatment is with splint or cast, with modified weight-bearing to prevent further displacement. Growth disturbance is unlikely, and healing is usually rapid. Physeal injuries of the ankle are the second most common growth plate injury following wrist fractures.

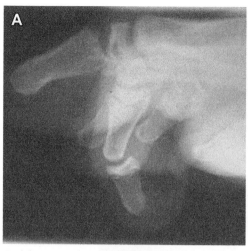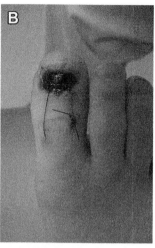

Fig. 3. (*A*) Type 1 physis fracture of the hallux. (*B*) Dorsal suspension technique to stabilize physeal fracture of the phalanx with large nonabsorbable suture through the nail bed and the extensor tendon. This technique is done using digital local anesthesia in the clinic or emergency room setting, avoiding the need for pinning or admission for operation. Strong plantar periosteum aids in reduction following dorsal tension of the suture.

damage to the growth plate and the periosteum. Inability to reduce the fracture or persistent gap of the physis may indicate that the periosteum is interposed in the physis and is an indication for ORIF. The authors always recommend obtaining radiographs of the contralateral extremity for comparison of physeal thickness and normal anatomic landmarks. This can prove invaluable for guidance in anatomic reduction (**Figs. 4–7**).

Type 3

This fracture pattern consists of a transverse physeal slip with a vertical fracture through the epiphysis. This is an intra-articular fracture at higher risk for growth disruption and arthrosis. CT scans are recommended to identify displacement and to plan for reduction. As with all intra-articular fractures, ORIF for accurate anatomic alignment and stability is recommended followed by appropriate splintage. As discussed previously, stable fixation and early range of motion should be the goal, and excessive periods of immobilization should be avoided (**Fig. 8**).

Type 4

This fracture pattern is a transverse slip through the physis and vertical fracture through the metaphysis and epiphysis. The management of this fracture pattern and the associated risks are the same as for type 3. ORIF is usually needed for anatomic reduction followed by appropriate splintage. Careful radiographic monitoring should be pursued after injury to assess for growth interruption and progressive angular deformity, which are higher in this fracture type.

Type 5

This injury pattern involves a compressive crush of the physis caused by an axial load through the epiphysis. There is no transverse slip of the physis and no visible metaphysis or epiphysis fracture on radiograph. This compression injury has a high risk of

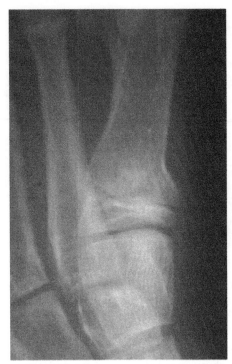

Fig. 4. Type 2 injury of the proximal first metatarsal. Note the displacement of the physis with fracture through the metaphysis.

growth interruption because of direct damage to the physeal cells. Treatment includes protected weight bearing and, most importantly, careful follow-up to identify growth interruption or progressive angular deformity.[4] Advanced techniques such as physeal debridement and reconstructive osteotomy may be required if progressive deformity results from growth interruption. The younger the patient is at the time of injury, the higher the risk of progressive deformity or limb length inequality. Older children have less time of growth remaining and therefore lower likelihood that progressive deformity will occur. Complications of this type and all other types of growth plate injury may result in the need for limb or bone segment lengthening in cases of significant deformity.

Type 6

One of the newer additions to the Salter-Harris classification is the Rang type 6 fracture. This fracture pattern follows a blunt trauma injury. The result is direct insult in which there is an injury to the perichondral ring with traumatic removal of physeal material. This injury is sometimes associated with lawnmower accidents, in which the rotary blade damages soft tissue and a portion of the peripheral physis.[5] Radiographic findings are widely varied but may be distinguished by the presence of a metaphyseal or epiphyseal fracture fragment within the periphery of the physis or obvious loss of the physeal and adjacent bone structures. Resulting callus from the bone and physeal injury makes the victim prone to asymmetric osseous bridging of the physis. This osseus bridging often leads to a progressive angular deformity due to partial physeal closure.[1]

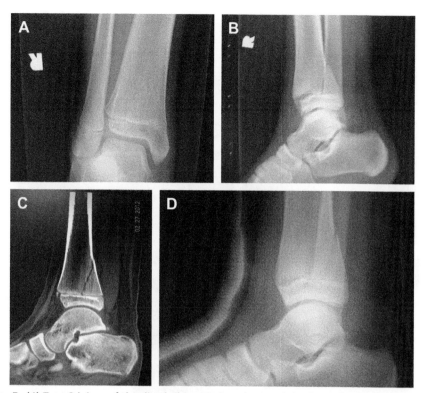

Fig. 5. (A) Type 2 injury of the distal tibia. AP view shows subtle signs of metaphyseal fracture. The slip of the physis is not visible on the AP view. These fractures are most common in the adolescent years. (B) Lateral view clearly showing the slip through the physis with displacement. (C) CT scan clarifies the fracture pattern and extent. Advanced imaging is recommended for most articular injuries and can aid in decision making for treatment. (D) Recommended treatment is closed reduction with casting. Thick periosteum in the pediatric patient aids in reduction and maintenance of fracture position with distraction and casting. Growth interruption is not common with this type of injury.

In cases of open trauma, treatment can be complicated due to the multiple variables. As with any open fracture, one should treat open pediatric fractures with careful systemic evaluation, appropriate antibiotics, and tetanus prophylaxis as indicated. This is followed by irrigation and meticulous debridement of devitalized tissue and foreign material.[6] Attention to stabilization of the soft tissue envelope, as well as the bone segments, is vital in open injuries. External fixation techniques can be invaluable to provide stability and allow access for debridement and reconstruction of both the soft tissue and the bone (**Fig. 9**).

TRANSITIONAL FRACTURES

The juvenile Tillaux and triplane fractures are classified as transitional fractures because of their occurrence in the period between adolescence and skeletal maturity, at which time the physis undergoes final closure. This transitional period is an approximately 18-month window when the distal tibia physis closes, and it usually starts at ages 12 to 14 years. The pattern of physeal closure proceeds from central, to

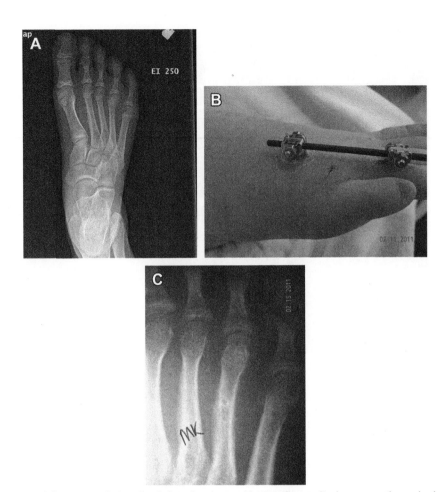

Fig. 6. (*A*) Type 2 of the distal fourth metatarsal. Significant displacement through the physis with subtle fracture of the metaphysis is evident. (*B*) External fixation was utilized for distraction and maintenance of the fracture position. External casting would not provide adequate stability in this location, and the fragments were too small for internal fixation. Fixator was minimally invasive and preserved the articular structures. (*C*) Result after reduction and healing of the fracture. The authors have used this technique successfully in a variety of pediatric peri-articular fractures including Frieberg infraction. Reduction and stabilization can be achieved with minimal additional soft tissue damage. In addition, the arthrodiastasis effect of the frame unloads the joint surfaces and the physis, allowing for consistent and rapid healing.

anteromedial, to posteromedial, and finally to lateral.[3] The process of medial physeal closure preceding lateral closure directly lends itself to the injury pattern observed during triplane and juvenile Tillaux fractures.

Juvenile Tillaux Fracture

The biplanar fracture of Tillaux is an avulsion fracture that occurs when the lateral aspect of the distal tibial epiphysis is pulled off by the intact distal tibiofibular ligaments. This mechanism of injury gives it a Salter-Harris type 3 fracture pattern. These

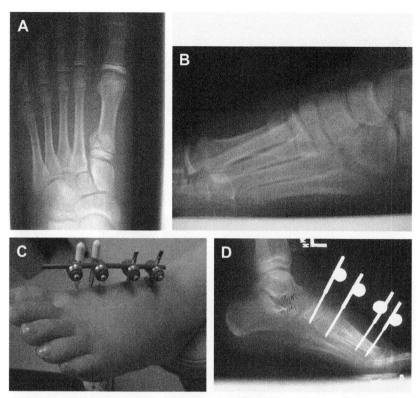

Fig. 7. (*A*) Type 2 of the proximal first metatarsal. Maintenance of reduction in this location is difficult with casting alone, and peri-articular location makes ORIF problematic. (*B*) Lateral view showing unacceptable displacement in the sagittal plane. (*C*) External fixation facilitates reduction and maintenance of position. Further damage to the physis, periosteal, and articular tissues is avoided. (*D*) Lateral view after reduction.

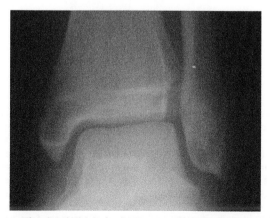

Fig. 8. Type 3 injury to the distal tibial physis. Degree of displacement is difficult to assess on plain film radiographs. CT scanning is recommended for all intra-articular fractures. This fracture pattern requires accurate reduction and stabilization, usually with ORIF.

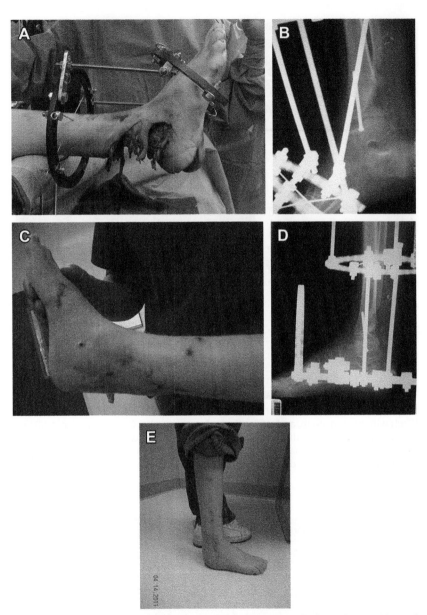

Fig. 9. (A) Lawn mover injury in 10-year-old child. Extensive soft tissue loss and bone frac-ture were sustained. External fixation provided stabilization of the soft tissue envelope and bone segments. The fixator facilitated access to tissues for wound care and soft tissue reconstruction. (B) Type 6 injury with extensive loss of the physeal tissues. (C) The original fixator was maintained throughout multiple operations for soft tissue reconstruction with ultimate free tissue transfer. The original fixator was removed after the soft tissues were healed. (D) Arthrodesis of the ankle and epiphsiodesis was required to halt progressive deformity from growth interruption of the physis and loss of the distal fibula. (E) Final result after limb salvage. Patient has partial sensation to the plantar foot and has stable well aligned ankle and foot with intact soft tissue envelope. Due to remaining growth potential at age 10, the patient may require limb lengthening in the future.

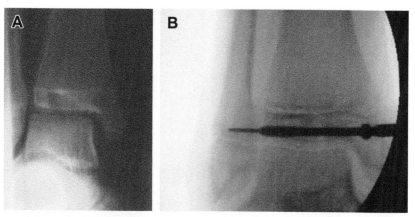

Fig. 10. (*A*) Juvenile Tillaux fracture. This represents a Salter Harris III fracture pattern in the transitional period of development. Because this fracture is intra-articular, careful assessment of displacement should be made with multiple radiographic views and CT scan. (*B*) Intraepiphyseal reduction technique utilizing cannulated screw. The fixation does not enter or cross the physis, so removal is typically not necessary.

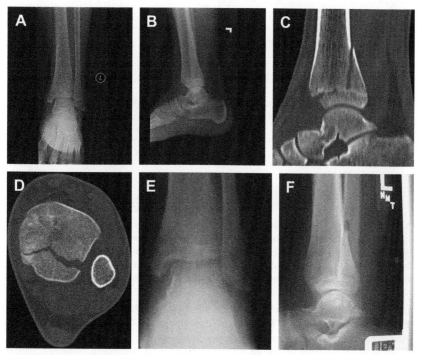

Fig. 11. (*A*) AP radiograph of triplane fracture. The type 3 fracture is easily visible. The type 2 metaphyseal fracture is present but is subtle on this view. (*B*) Lateral view showing typical physeal displacement and typical metaphyseal fracture orientation. (*C*) CT view showing sagittal displacement of the tibia. (*D*) Minimal displacement of the epiphysis fracture is noted on CT scan. (*E, F*) Closed reduction under general anesthesia was accomplished, and a long leg cast was placed to maintain reduction. Because minimal epiphysis displacement was present, closed reduction resulted in good position and healing.

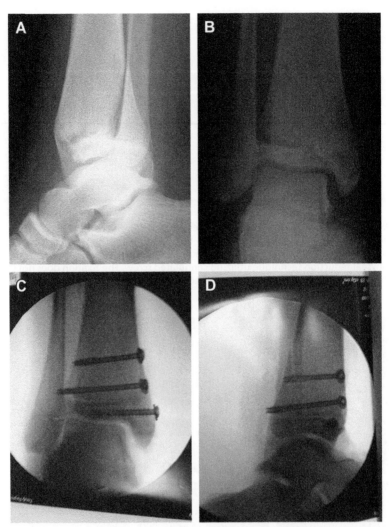

Fig. 12. (*A*) Lateral view of displaced triplane fracture. The transverse plane physeal slip and the frontal plane metaphysis fracture are visible. (*B*) AP view showing the third plane of injury in the sagittal plane. (*C, D*) Open reduction and internal fixation using recommended fixation placement to stabilize all 3 components of the fracture. Stable fixation will allow for early range of motion to preserve joint function and speed rehabilitation.

fractures are comparable in location to the adult Tillaux Chaput fracture, which shares a similar mechanism of injury. The fracture itself is not full-thickness anterior to posterior, and it occurs during the transitional period when only the lateral physis has yet to fuse.[3] In a retrospective study of 237 pediatric ankle fractures, Spiegel and colleagues[7] reported that only 6 (2.5%) were juvenile Tillaux fracture types. These cases occurred at an average patient age of 13 years and 5 months.

The overall outcome after juvenile Tillaux fractures is good, with rare occurrences of angular deformity and minimal risks of growth discrepancy. However, the risk for osteoarthritis is high if articular step-off remains after treatment; therefore, the clinician should carefully evaluate the amount of displacement before and after reduction.[3]

Nondisplaced and minimally displaced fractures may be treated with immobilization in a long or short leg cast. However, ORIF is often necessary because of the intra- articular nature of the fracture. It is important to remember that compressive fixation elements used during ORIF should not enter or cross the physis. Postoperatively, the patient should remain nonweight-bearing in a cast for 3 weeks followed by an additional 3 weeks in a walking cast or brace. A stable fracture construct will allow for early range of motion, which is desirable to preserve articular soft tissue function (**Fig. 10**).

Triplane Fracture

Consistent with transitional fractures, the triplane fracture occurs as a result of relative weakness of the anterolateral tibial physis. Typically, triplane fractures occur approximately 1 year later in boys when compared with girls. As with all transitional fractures, this is attributed to the age difference of physis closure. The injury is a result of external rotation forces, and there is an associated fibular fracture seen in up to 50% of cases.[8] As the name would suggest, the triplane fracture always contains a fracture element in each of the 3 cardinal body planes, and fractures are evident in the epiphysis, metaphysis, and the physis.[9]

When evaluating these fractures on plain film, it is important to assess multiple views. The triplane fracture may appear as a type 3 fracture or Tillaux fracture on the anterior-posterior (AP) view. However, evaluation of additional views will reveal a type 2 fracture on the lateral view. The transverse component of the fracture connects the sagittal and coronal fractures as it traverses the physis.[3]

When planning for treatment, these injuries must have accurate radiographic diagnosis. This is optimally performed with a CT scan using multiplanar reconstructions for more accurate assessment of the amount of displacement and the extension of fracture lines.[10] Treatment of a displaced epiphyseal fracture requires ORIF. The postreduction regimen follows that of type 3 and 4 fractures. There is little risk of subsequent growth abnormality or progressive angulation from this fracture, because physiologic closure is already occurring. Additionally, little growth remains at this anatomic site (**Figs. 11** and **12**).

SUMMARY

Because of the unique histologic and mechanical properties of the pediatric skeletal and physiology of the physis, pediatric growth plate fractures cause pose a challenge for the treating physician. It is imperative that these characteristics be taken into account and the physician have a thorough understanding of the pediatric bone and healing properties, which vary significantly from mature bone. With a thorough understanding, clearly stated goals and limitations of treatment explained to the patient and parents, and institution of appropriate treatment, the care of these patients can be extremely rewarding.

REFERENCES

1. DeValentine S. Foot and ankle disorders in children. New York: Churchill Livingstone; 1992.
2. Podeszwa DA, Mubarak SJ. Physeal fractures of the distal tibia and fibula (Salter-Harris type I, II, III, and IV fractures). J Pediatr Orthop 2012;32:S62–8.
3. Bible JE, Smith BG. Ankle fractures in children and adolescents. Techniques in Orthopaedics 2009;24:211–9.
4. Harris JH. Physeal injuries. Contemp Diagn Radiol 2005;28:1–5.

5. Nugent N, Lynch J, O'Shaughnessy M, et al. Lawnmower injuries in children. Eur J Emerg Med 2006;13:286–9.
6. Blackburn EW, Aronsson DD, Rubright JH, et al. Ankle fractures in children. J Bone Joint Surg Am 2012;94:1234–44.
7. Spiegel PG, Cooperman DR, Laros GS. Epiphyseal fractures of the distal ends of the tibia and fibula. A retrospective study of two hundred and thirty-seven cases in children. J Bone Joint Surg Am 1978;60:1046–50.
8. Ertl JP, Barrack RL, Alexander AH, et al. Triplane fracture of the distal tibial epiphysis. Long-term follow-up. J Bone Joint Surg Am 1988;70:967–76.
9. Brown SD, Kasser JR, Zurakowski D, et al. Analysis of 51 tibial triplane fractures using CT with multiplanar reconstruction. AJR Am J Roentgenol 2004;183(5):1489–95.
10. Ho-Fung V, Pollock A. Triplane fracture. Pediatr Emerg Care 2011;27:70–2.

Current Concepts and Techniques in Foot and Ankle Surgery

Simultaneous Surgical Repair of a Tibialis Anterior Tendon Rupture and Diabetic Charcot Neuroarthropathy of the Midfoot
A Case Report

John J. Stapleton, DPM[a,b,*]

KEYWORDS

- Tendon rupture • Tibialis anterior tendon • Charcot foot • Charcot neuroarthropathy
- Diabetes mellitus

KEY POINTS

- Tibialis anterior tendon rupture with diabetic Charcot neuroarthropathy of the midfoot was successfully treated with a tendon transfer and a medical column arthrodesis.
- Tendon ruptures have been associated in patients with diabetes mellitus.
- External fixation can play a pivotal role in this clinical presentation.

Rupture of the tibialis anterior (TA) tendon has been reported in the literature, with the most common findings associated with an acute trauma on forced plantarflexion of the foot and ankle and/or with a chronic tendinous degenerative process.[1–6] Diabetes mellitus has also been linked to tendon thickening, tendinosis, and spontaneous rupture[7] and previously reported with a spontaneous TA rupture in a diabetic patient.[8] In this case report, the author presents a surgical repair to address a TA tendon rupture in a diabetic patient with a Charcot neuroarthropathy (CN) midfoot deformity.

CASE REPORT

A 58-year old man well known to the author's practice with a history of diabetes mellitus, peripheral neuropathy, and multiple medical co-morbidities was followed for the contralateral left foot CN that was surgically repaired with a midfoot osteotomy, acute deformity correction, and external fixation 3-years prior to his clinical presentation of

[a] Foot and Ankle Surgery, VSAS Orthopaedics, Lehigh Valley Hospital, 1250 South Cedar Crest Boulevard, Suite # 110, Allentown, PA 18103, USA; [b] Penn State College of Medicine, 500 University Drive, Hershey, PA 17033, USA
* Corresponding author.
E-mail address: jostaple@hotmail.com

the symptomatic right foot. After the surgical reconstruction of the left foot, the patient had resumed functional ambulation with extradepth shoe gear and custom inlays and without any evidence of CN to the right foot (**Fig. 1**). At the new presentation, the patient reported a history of an atraumatic onset of swelling and warmth to the right foot and ankle for a few months duration. Besides the right lower extremity edema, the patient reported no pain to the affected foot and ankle, which presented with a pre-ulcerative lesion on the plantar aspect of the medial cuneiform. The patient's vascular examination revealed nonbounding palpable dorsalis and posterior tibial artery pulses, and instability of the right tarsometatarsal joint was apparent on musculoskeletal examination. An equinus contracture at the right ankle was evident with the knee extended and flexed. In addition, a palpable soft tissue mass 5 to 6 cm proximal to the medial cuneiform insertion of the TA tendon was evident, and the patient was unable to simultaneously dorsiflex and invert the foot against resistance of gravity. Plain foot radiographs demonstrated a neuropathic right foot Lisfranc fracture–dislocation with associated collapse of the medial longitudinal arch (**Fig. 2**). Subsequent magnetic resonance imaging revealed a complete rupture of the TA tendon with retraction to the level of the ankle joint along with CN changes involving the midfoot. Surgical treatment options were discussed with the patient, emphasizing the severity and the progressive nature of the deformity and risk for ulceration. Further conservative treatment options were also discussed with the patient, including the prolonged use of a Charcot-restrained orthotic walker, but the patient elected for surgical repair, with the most influencing factor being his successful surgical outcome to the contralateral left foot.

SURGICAL TECHNIQUE

Definitive repair of the CN midfoot deformity and TA tendon rupture was performed with the patient under general anesthesia in the supine position and the utilization of a thigh tourniquet. A percutaneous triple hemisection tendo-Achilles lengthening

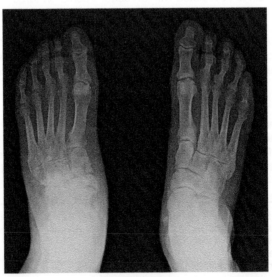

Fig. 1. Anteroposterior radiograph of the right foot 3 years prior to current presentation demonstrated no evidence of CN. Note that the patient had a healed midfoot osteotomy to address a CN midfoot deformity to the contralateral left foot at that time.

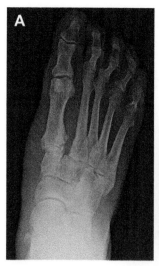
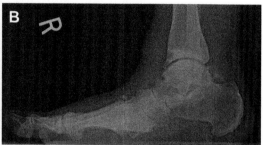

Fig. 2. (*A*) Anteroposterior and (*B*) lateral radiographs of the right foot demonstrating CN involving the midfoot with fracture, subluxation, and associated collapse.

(TAL) and a total of 3 incisions were utilized for surgical exposure, including the tendon transfer and medial column arthrodesis procedures (**Fig. 3**). The initial part of the surgery started with performing a percutaneous TAL to address the equinus contracture. Next, the surgical exposure of the medial column was performed, and realignment was achieved by performing a medial column arthrodesis involving the medial tarsometatarsal joint, navicular–cuneiform joints, and talonavicular joint. After the joints were prepared and aligned for arthrodesis, a Steinmann pin was utilized to initially stabilize the medial column. Attention was then directed to harvest the extensor hallucis longus (EHL) tendon at the level just proximal to the interphalangeal joint (IPJ) of the hallux and with the extensor hallucis brevis being sutured to the distal stump of the EHL tendon. Next, crossed Kirschner wires were inserted across the IPJ to prevent flexion and contracture of the right hallux. Surgical dissection was then continued at the anterior aspect of the ankle joint to expose the ruptured TA tendon. The affected tendon displayed significant tendinosis, and its degenerate portion was excised as necessary. Muscle excursion of the TA tendon was also evident upon exposure at the ankle level. Next, a 5 mm drill hole was placed into the dorsal and medial aspect of the medial cuneiform to allow passage of the EHL tendon followed by a pulvertaft weave of the EHL through the proximal portion of the TA tendon. Distally, the EHL was transferred through the osseous tunnel in the medial cuneiform and then sutured back onto itself under maximum tension while the foot was held in a dorsiflexed position (**Fig. 4**). At the end of previously mentioned surgical procedures, the tourniquet was then deflated; hemostasis was achieved, and wound closure was performed in the usual manner and prior to application of the circular external fixator (**Fig. 5**). Next, smooth transosseous wires and half pins were inserted in anatomic safe zones to stabilize the circular external fixator to the right lower extremity. Compression of the medial column arthrodesis site(s) was performed with a bent wire tensioning technique (**Fig. 6**). The patient was kept nonweight bearing with the circular external fixator retained for 10 weeks. After removal of the external fixator, the patient was placed into a nonweight-bearing cast for 2 weeks followed by a walking cast for an additional 2 weeks. The patient resumed functional ambulation with accommodative shoe gear

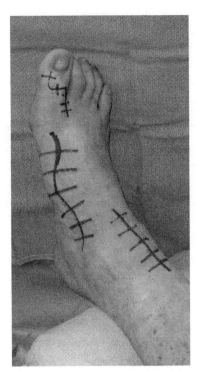

Fig. 3. Clinical picture of the right foot demonstrating incision placement utilized to perform a simultaneous medial column arthrodesis and extensor hallucis longus tendon transfer to address the tibialis anterior tendon rupture.

and adequate dorsiflexion and inversion muscle strength without any evidence of a foot drop or need for an ankle foot orthosis. At approximately 6 months postoperatively, plain foot radiographs revealed successful arthrodesis of the medial column (**Fig. 7**).

A **B**

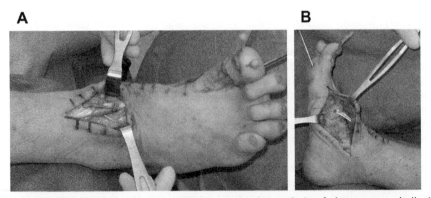

Fig. 4. (*A*) Clinical picture demonstrating a proximal tenodesis of the extensor hallucis longus and tibialis anterior tendon utilizing a pulvertaft weave technique. (*B*) Attachment of the extensor hallucis longus tendon was performed through an osseous tunnel placed in the medial cuneiform.

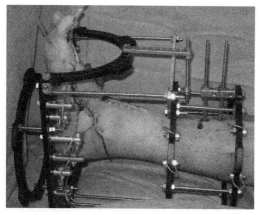

Fig. 5. Clinical picture demonstrating the utilization of a circular external fixator to achieve compression and stability of the medial column arthrodesis sites while preventing plantar-flexion of the foot and minimizing injury at the tendon transfer/repair junctions.

DISCUSSION

This case report has demonstrated a surgical repair of TA rupture with a diabetic CN midfoot deformity that was addressed with a medial column arthrodesis to provide stability and realignment of the medial longitudinal arch and an EHL tendon transfer, because a primary repair was not feasible given the size of the rupture gap, suspected rupture chronicity, and degenerative condition of the tendon. A proximal tenodesis of the EHL and TA tendon was performed, because the TA muscle displayed adequate excursion intraoperatively. In addition, an osseous tunnel was utilized for further strength and reconstruction to the normal insertion of the TA tendon. An external

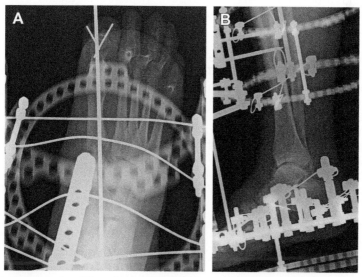

Fig. 6. Anteroposterior (*A*) and lateral (*B*) radiographs of the right foot demonstrating realignment and compression of the medial column arthrodesis sites.

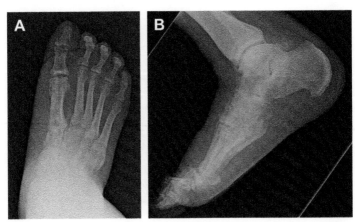

Fig. 7. (*A*) Anteroposterior and (*B*) lateral radiographs of the right foot at approximately 6 months postoperatively, demonstrating successful arthrodesis and deformity correction.

fixation device was utilized to achieve compression of the medial column arthrodesis sites where internal fixation might have interfered with the EHL tendon transfer to the medial cuneiform. In conclusion, this case report has shown a unique clinical presentation that might raise a higher index of suspicion for tendon ruptures that may coexist with the diabetic CN.

REFERENCES

1. Kausch T, Rutt J. Subcutaneous rupture of the tibialis anterior tendon: review of literature and a case report. Arch Orthop Trauma Surg 1998;117:290–3.
2. Ouzounian TJ, Anderson R. Anterior tibial tendon rupture. Foot Ankle Int 1995; 167:406–10.
3. Anagnostakos K, Bachelier F, Furst OA, et al. Rupture of the anterior tibial tendon, three clinical cases, anatomic study, and review of the literature. Foot Ankle Int 2006;27:330–9.
4. Patten A, Pun WK. Spontaneous rupture of the tibialis anterior tendon: a case report and review of the literature. Foot Ankle Int 2000;218:697–700.
5. Omari AM, Lee AS, Parsons SW. The Clinical presentation of chronic tibialis anterior insufficiency. Foot Ankle Surg 1999;54:251–6.
6. Moyer J, Kosanovich R. Anterior tibial tendon injuries. Clin Podiatr Med Surg 2002;19:433–40.
7. Ramirez LC, Raskin P. Diabetic foot tendinopathy: abnormalities in the flexor plantar tendons in patients with diabetes mellitus. J Diabet Complications 1998;126:337–9.
8. DiDomenico LA, Williams K, Petrolla AF. Spontaneous rupture of the anterior tibial tendon in a diabetic patient: results of operative treatment. Foot Ankle Surg 2008; 45:463–7.

Erratum

An error was made in the April 2013 issue of *Clinics in Podiatric Medicine and Surgery*. On page 251, the article "Concomitant Osteomyelitis and Avascular Necrosis of the Talus Treated with Talectomy and Tibiocalcaneal Arthrodesis" by Drs. John J. Stapleton and Thomas Zgonis was printed with the wrong abstract. The correct abstract is as follows:

Surgical management of post-traumatic avascular necrosis and/or diabetic Charcot neuroarthropathy complications of the talus present with a great challenge to the treating physician. The incidence of avascular necrosis from a complex talus fracture is relatively high and can become more problematic when associated with infection, nonunion, and structural collapse. Post-traumatic reconstruction of high energy talus injuries is commonly associated with a poor soft tissue envelope limiting the surgeon to utilize intramedullary nails or external fixation to achieve a salvage arthrodesis. Similarly, avascular necrosis of the talus with concomitant osteomyelitis and large soft tissue defect can be found in the diabetic population with Charcot neuroarthropathy of the hindfoot and ankle. The goal of this article is to overview the utilization of circular external fixation combined with adequate surgical debridement and talectomy to perform a single or multiple staged tibiocalcaneal arthrodesis and how this may differ depending on the clinical presentation.

Clin Podiatr Med Surg 30 (2013) 605
http://dx.doi.org/10.1016/j.cpm.2013.08.003
0891-8422/13/$ – see front matter © 2013 Elsevier Inc. All rights reserved.

podiatric.theclinics.com

Erratum

Errors were made in the October 2012 issue of *Clinics in Podiatric Medicine and Surgery*. On page 549, in the article the article "Total Ankle Replacement: A Historical Perspective" by Dr. Benjamin D. Overley, in the second sentence of the first paragraph, "Hintermann" was intended to be "Saltzman" with reference 82 cited. In the next sentence "Barg and Hintermann Study" was intended to be the "Waters Study": Waters RL, Barnes G, Husserl T, Comparable energy expenditure after arthrodesis of the hip and ankle. JBJS Am 1988;70(7):1032–7.

On page 558, Figures 17 and 18 are incorrectly identified and are actually photos of the Hintegra Total Ankle device.

Clin Podiatr Med Surg 30 (2013) 607
http://dx.doi.org/10.1016/j.cpm.2013.08.004
podiatric.theclinics.com

Index

Note: Page numbers of article titles are in **boldface** type.

A

Abductor hallucis tendon procedures, for hallux varus, 536–537
Acetabular disorders, intoeing in, 551–553
Akron dome osteotomy, for cavus deformities, 547
Anchor sign, 466
Ankle equinus, 463–464, 474–475, 495
Anterior drawer test, 467, 469
Antibiotics, for calcaneal osteomyelitis, 509
Apophysitis, calcaneal, 503–505
Apprehension test, patellar, 467
Arch, abnormally high, 474–475
ARM method, for metatarsus adductus, 469
Arm swing, in gait, 462

B

Babinski sign, 476
Barlow sign, 466, 468
Bone cysts, calcaneal, 505–506
Brachymetatarsia, 482
Buckle fractures, 594
Bunionectomy, for hallux valgus, 487

C

Calcaneal stance position, 464–465
Calcaneus
    anatomy of, 503
    apophysitis of, 503–505
    fractures of, 506–507
    osteomyelitis of, 507–509
    retained foreign body in, 509
Casting
    for clubfoot, 515–516
    for first ray deformities, 495
    for growth plate fractures, 588
    for metatarsus adductus, 539–540
    for talipes equinovarus, 543–544
    for tibial torsion, 551
Cavus foot
    evaluation of, 474–475
    intoeing in, 544–547

Clin Podiatr Med Surg 30 (2013) 609–616
http://dx.doi.org/10.1016/S0891-8422(13)00096-7
0891-8422/13/$ – see front matter © 2013 Elsevier Inc. All rights reserved.

Cellulitis, from retained foreign body, 509
Center of gravity, in gait, 462–463
Cerebral palsy
    femoral anteversion in, 555–556, 560–561
    first ray deformities in, 493
Charcot neuroarthropathy, tibialis anterior tendon rupture in, **599–604**
Charcot-Marie-Tooth syndrome, cavus deformities in, 545
Closed reduction, for growth plate fractures, 587–588
Closing osteotomy, for metatarsus adductus, 539–540
Clubfoot
    causes of, 470
    evaluation of, 470–471
    neglected and relapsed, **513–530**
        author's preferences for, 523–525
        bone procedures for, 516–519
        definition of, 513–515
        external fixation for, 519–523
        Ponseti method for, 513–514, 523
        soft tissue procedures for, 515–516
    staging of, 470–471
Cognitive disability, first ray deformities with, 499–500
Cole procedure, for cavus deformities, 547
Coleman block test, 475
Coxa vara, 462
Cysts, calcaneal, 505–506

D

Diabetic foot, tibialis anterior tendon rupture in, **599–604**
Dorsalis pedis pulse, 476
Double heel rise test, 472–473
Dwyer osteotomy, for clubfoot, 518
Dyer and Davis scoring system, for clubfoot, 470–471

E

Evans osteotomy, for clubfoot, 517
Examination, **461–478**
    non–weight-bearing, 465–469
    of foot deformities, 469–476
    weight-bearing, 461–465
External fixation
    for clubfoot, 519–523
    for growth plate fractures, 591–594
Extraosseus talotarsal stabilization devices, for talometatarsal joint displacement, 576–578

F

Femoral anteversion, intoeing in, 554–561
Femoral anteversion (antetorsion, medial femoral torsion), intoeing in, 554–561

Femoral head, abnormalities of, 553
Femur, angle of, 465–466
First ray deformities, **491–501**
    age-related treatment of, 494–500
    causes of, 491–493
Flatfoot
    anatomy of, 568
    evaluation of, 571–572
    flexible, evaluation of, 472–473
    pathophysiology of, 568–569
    radiography for, 572–573
    rigid, evaluation of, 471
    signs and symptoms of, 570–571
    treatment of, 573–578
Fluoroscopy, for talotarsal joint displacement, 572–573
Footwear
    for first ray deformities, 494–499
    tarsotarsal joint displacement clues in, 570–571
Forefoot pathology, **479–490**
    brachymetatarsia, 482
    hallux valgus, 472–473, 486–488
    macrodactyly, 481
    metatarsal, 482–486
    polydactyly, 479–481
    syndactyly, 481–482
    varus deformity, 473–474
Foreign body, retained in heel, 509
Fractures
    calcaneal, 506–507
    growth plate, **583–598**
        classification of, 587–591
        healing of, 583–584
        histologic considerations in, 584–586
        open, 590–591
        remodeling in, 586
        transitional, 591–597
        treatment of, 586–597
    metatarsal, 482–484
    phalangeal, 484
Freiberg disease, 485–486

G

Gait, evaluation of, 461–465
Gait analysis, for tarsotarsal joint displacement, 572
Galeazzi sign, 466
Genu recurvatum, 464
Genu valgum, 464
Genu varum, 464
"Growing pains," in tarsotarsal joint displacement, 570
Growth plate fractures. See Fractures, growth plate.

H

Hallux valgus, 472–473, 486–488
   causes of, 491–493
   treatment of, 494–500
Hallux varus, intoeing in, 534–537
Head position, evaluation of, 462
Head-neck-greater trochanter axis, 552–554
Heel pain, **503–511**
   anatomic considerations in, 503
   in bone tumors, 505–506
   in fractures, 506–507
   in osteomyelitis, 507–509
   in Sever disease, 503–505
   retained foreign body causing, 509
Heyman-Herndon-Strong procedure, for metatarsus adductus, 539
Hip, orthopedic examination of, 465–466
Hubscher maneuver, 472–474
Hypermobility, in hallux abducto valgus, 472–473

I

Ilizarov external fixation, for clubfoot, 519–523
Immobilization, for Iselin's disease, 485
Internal fixation, for growth plate fractures, 587, 589–591
Intoeing, **531–565**
   age of onset of, 533
   causes of, 532–533
   definition of, 532
   in acetabular disorders, 551–553
   in cavus deformity, 544–547
   in hallux varus, 533–537
   in metatarsus adductus, 538–540
   in talipes equinovarus, 540–544
   in tibial torsion, 547–551
   treatment of, 522–523
Iselin's disease, 484–485

J

Jack, toe test of, 472–474
Jendrassik maneuver, 476

K

Knee
   orthopedic examination of, 466–467, 469
   position of, evaluation of, 462
Kyphosis, 462

L

Lachmann test, 467, 469
Lawrence classification, of metatarsal base fractures, 484

Lichtblau procedure, for hallux varus, 536–537
Limb length discrepancy, 462
Lipomas, calcaneal, 505–506
Longitudinal epiphyseal bracket, 486, 537

M

Macrodactyly, 481
Magnetic resonance imaging, for bone tumors, 506
Medial capsulorraphy, for first ray deformities, 497
Metatarsal(s)
    fractures of, 482–484
    Freiberg disease of, 485–486
    Iselin's disease of, 484–485
    longitudinal epiphyseal bracket in, 486
    shortening of, 482
Metatarsus adductus
    causes of, 491–493
    evaluation of, 469–470
    intoeing in, 538–540
    treatment of, 494–500
Midfoot osteotomy, for clubfoot, 520
Musculoskeletal examination, 478

N

Neurologic disorders
    cavus deformities in, 545
    femoral anteversion in, 555–556
    gait in, 462
Neurologic examination, 475–476

O

Opening wedge osteotomy, for metatarsus adductus, 539–540
Orthosis
    for first ray deformities, 496–499
    for Freiberg disease, 485–486
    for talotarsal joint displacement, 574–575
Ortolani sign, 466
Osteochondral autograft transfer system, for Freiberg disease, 485–486
Osteochondrosis, in Freiberg disease, 485–486
Osteoid osteomas, calcaneal, 505–506
Osteomyelitis, calcaneal, 507–509
Osteotomy
    for cavus deformities, 547
    for clubfoot, 517–520
    for femoral anteversion, 560
    for metatarsus adductus, 539–540
    for polydactyly, 481
    for tibial torsion, 551

P

Pain, heel, **503–511**
Pain management
    for bone tumors, 505–506
    for first ray deformities, 496–500
    for Sever disease, 505
Patella, orthopedic examination of, 466–467
Pediatric foot deformities
    clubfoot. *See* Clubfoot.
    examination for, **461–478**
    first ray, **491–501**
    forefoot, **479–490**
    growth plate fractures and, **583–598**
    heel pain in, **503–511**
    intoeing, **531–565**
    pes planovalgus, **567–581**
Pelvic position, evaluation of, 462
Pelvic tilt, 462
Pes cavus
    evaluation of, 474–475
    intoeing in, 544–547
Pes planovalgus. *See* Flatfoot.
Phalanges, fractures of, 484
Physeal injuries. *See* Fractures, growth plate.
Physical therapy
    for clubfoot, 516
    for femoral anteversion, 560
Pirani score, for clubfoot, 471
Plantar fascia release, for clubfoot, 522
Polydactyly, 479–481
Polysyndactyly, 481–482
Ponseti method, 513–514, 523, 543–544
Posterior drawer test, 469
Pronation, excessive, first ray deformities and, 491–501
Pseudoequinus, 475
Pulses, evaluation of, 476

R

Radiography
    for calcaneal fracture, 507
    for calcaneal osteomyelitis, 509
    for growth plate fractures, 586–587
    for Sever disease, 504–505
    for talotarsal joint displacement, 572–573
Remodeling, of growth plate fractures, 586
Ryder maneuver, 556
Ryder test, 465–466

S

Salter-Harris classification, of fractures, 587–591
Scoliosis, 462, 474–475
Serial casting
  for clubfoot, 515–516
  for metatarsus adductus, 539–540
  for talipes equinovarus, 543–544
Sever disease, 503–505
Shoulder position, evaluation of, 462
Silfverskiöld test, 464
Skewfoot, 540
Slipped capital femoral epiphysis, 553
Soft tissue balancing, for first ray deformities, 497
Soft tissue procedures, for clubfoot, 515–516
"Squinting patella sign," in femoral anteversion, 556
Stress inversion test, 469
Supramalleolar osteotomy, for clubfoot, 520
Syndactyly, 481–482
Syringomyelia, cavus deformities in, 545

T

Talectomy, for clubfoot, 519
Talipes equinovarus, intoeing in, 540–544
Talotarsal joint displacement, **567–581**
  anatomy of, 568
  evaluation of, 571–572
  pathophysiology of, 568–569
  radiography for, 572–573
  signs and symptoms of, 570–571
  treatment of, 573–578
Tarsal coalition
  rigid flatfoot for, 471
  talotarsal joint displacement and, 573
Tarsometatarsal release, for metatarsus adductus, 539
Taylor Spatial Frame, for clubfoot, 519–523
Television-sitting position, femoral anteversion in, 555
Tendon reflexes, evaluation of, 475–476
Tetanus prophylaxis, for retained foreign body, 509
Thomas test, 464
Thompson and Simons classification, for talipes equinovarus, 541–543
Tibial torsion, 464–465, 547–551
Tibialis anterior tendon
  rupture of, in diabetic foot, **599–604**
  transfer of, for clubfoot, 515–516
Tillaux fractures, juvenile, 591, 595–597
Toe(s)
  fused together (syndactyly), 481–482
  overgrowth of (macrodactyly), 481

Toe(s) (*continued*)
　supernumerary (polydactyly), 479–481
Toe test of Jack, 472–474
Toe walking, 463–464
Toeing-in, 462
Toe-walking, in tarsotarsal joint displacement, 572
"Too many toes" sign, in tarsotarsal joint displacement, 572
Torsional profile, 533
Torus fractures, 594
Traction epiphysitis, 484–485
Trendelenburg gait, 462
Triplane fractures, 591–592, 597
Trunk position, evaluation of, 462
Tumors, calcaneal, 505–506

U

U osteotomy, for clubfoot, 519–520
Unicameral bone cysts, calcaneal, 505–506

V

V osteotomy, for clubfoot, 520
Valgus deformity
　hallux, 472–473
　knee, 464
Varus deformity, forefoot, 473–474
Vascular examination, 476

W

W-sitting position, femoral anteversion in, 555

United States Postal Service
Statement of Ownership, Management, and Circulation
(All Periodicals Publications Except Requestor Publications)

1. Publication Title	2. Publication Number	3. Filing Date
Clinics in Podiatric Medicine & Surgery	0 0 0 - 7 0 7	9/14/13

4. Issue Frequency	5. Number of Issues Published Annually	6. Annual Subscription Price
Jan, Apr, Jul, Oct	4	$292.00

7. Complete Mailing Address of Known Office of Publication (Not printer) (Street, city, county, state, and ZIP+4®)

Elsevier Inc.
360 Park Avenue South
New York, NY 10010-1710

Contact Person
Stephen R. Bushing

Telephone (Include area code)
215-239-3688

8. Complete Mailing Address of Headquarters or General Business Office of Publisher (Not printer)

Elsevier Inc., 360 Park Avenue South, New York, NY 10010-1710

9. Full Names and Complete Mailing Addresses of Publisher, Editor, and Managing Editor (Do not leave blank)

Publisher (Name and complete mailing address)

Linda Belfus, Elsevier, Inc., 1600 John F. Kennedy Blvd. Suite 1800, Philadelphia, PA 19103-2899

Editor (Name and complete mailing address)

Patrick Manley, Elsevier, Inc., 1600 John F. Kennedy Blvd. Suite 1800, Philadelphia, PA 19103-2899

Managing Editor (Name and complete mailing address)

Barbara Cohen - Kligerman, Elsevier, Inc., 1600 John F. Kennedy Blvd. Suite 1800, Philadelphia, PA 19103-2899

10. Owner (Do not leave blank. If the publication is owned by a corporation, give the name and address of the corporation immediately followed by the names and addresses of all stockholders owning or holding 1 percent or more of the total amount of stock. If not owned by a corporation, give the names and addresses of the individual owners. If owned by a partnership or other unincorporated firm, give its name and address as well as those of each individual owner. If the publication is published by a nonprofit organization, give its name and address.)

Full Name	Complete Mailing Address
Wholly owned subsidiary of	1600 John F. Kennedy Blvd., Ste. 1800
Reed/Elsevier, US holdings	Philadelphia, PA 19103-2899

11. Known Bondholders, Mortgagees, and Other Security Holders Owning or Holding 1 Percent or More of Total Amount of Bonds, Mortgages, or Other Securities. If none, check box ☐ None

Full Name	Complete Mailing Address
N/A	

12. Tax Status (For completion by nonprofit organizations authorized to mail at nonprofit rates) (Check one)
The purpose, function, and nonprofit status of this organization and the exempt status for federal income tax purposes:
☐ Has Not Changed During Preceding 12 Months
☐ Has Changed During Preceding 12 Months (Publisher must submit explanation of change with this statement)

PS Form 3526, September 2007 (Page 1 of 3 (Instructions Page 3)) PSN 7530-01-000-9931 PRIVACY NOTICE: See our Privacy policy in www.usps.com

---

13. Publication Title	14. Issue Date for Circulation Data Below
Clinics in Podiatric Medicine & Surgery	July 2013

15. Extent and Nature of Circulation		Average No. Copies Each Issue During Preceding 12 Months	No. Copies of Single Issue Published Nearest to Filing Date
a. Total Number of Copies (Net press run)		623	574
b. Paid Circulation (By Mail and Outside the Mail)	(1) Mailed Outside-County Paid Subscriptions Stated on PS Form 3541. (Include paid distribution above nominal rate, advertiser's proof copies, and exchange copies)	424	373
	(2) Mailed In-County Paid Subscriptions Stated on PS Form 3541 (Include paid distribution above nominal rate, advertiser's proof copies, and exchange copies)		
	(3) Paid Distribution Outside the Mails Including Sales Through Dealers and Carriers, Street Vendors, Counter Sales, and Other Paid Distribution Outside USPS®	40	42
	(4) Paid Distribution by Other Classes Mailed Through the USPS (e.g. First-Class Mail®)		
c. Total Paid Distribution (Sum of 15b (1), (2), (3), and (4))	▶	464	415
d. Free or Nominal Rate Distribution (By Mail and Outside the Mail)	(1) Free or Nominal Rate Outside-County Copies Included on PS Form 3541	71	71
	(2) Free or Nominal Rate In-County Copies Included on PS Form 3541		
	(3) Free or Nominal Rate Copies Mailed at Other Classes Through the USPS (e.g. First-Class Mail)		
	(4) Free or Nominal Rate Distribution Outside the Mail (Carriers or other means)		
e. Total Free or Nominal Rate Distribution (Sum of 15d (1), (2), (3) and (4))	▶	71	71
f. Total Distribution (Sum of 15c and 15e)	▶	535	486
g. Copies not Distributed (See instructions to publishers #4 (page #3))	▶	88	88
h. Total (Sum of 15f and g)	▶	623	574
i. Percent Paid (15c divided by 15f times 100)		86.73%	85.39%

16. Publication of Statement of Ownership

☐ If the publication is a general publication, publication of this statement is required. Will be printed in the October 2013 issue of this publication. ☐ Publication not required

17. Signature and Title of Editor, Publisher, Business Manager, or Owner

Stephen R. Bushing — Inventory/Distribution Coordinator

Date: September 14, 2013

I certify that all information furnished on this form is true and complete. I understand that anyone who furnishes false or misleading information on this form or who omits material or information requested on the form may be subject to criminal sanctions (including fines and imprisonment) and/or civil sanctions (including civil penalties).

PS Form 3526, September 2007 (Page 2 of 3)

Moving?

Make sure your subscription moves with you!

To notify us of your new address, find your **Clinics Account Number** (located on your mailing label above your name), and contact customer service at:

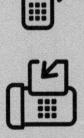

Email: journalscustomerservice-usa@elsevier.com

800-654-2452 (subscribers in the U.S. & Canada)
314-447-8871 (subscribers outside of the U.S. & Canada)

Fax number: 314-447-8029

Elsevier Health Sciences Division
Subscription Customer Service
3251 Riverport Lane
Maryland Heights, MO 63043

*To ensure uninterrupted delivery of your subscription, please notify us at least 4 weeks in advance of move.

Printed and bound by CPI Group (UK) Ltd, Croydon, CR0 4YY

03/10/2024

01040478-0016